ATI TEAS

High-Yield Practice for the New ATI TEAS

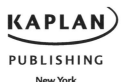

KAPLAN

PUBLISHING

New York

Special thanks to the team that made this book possible: Gina Allison, Erika Blumenthal, Joel Boyce, Chanti Burnette, Matthew Callan, Irene Cheung, Dorothy Cummings, Lola Dart, Marilyn Engle, Paula Fleming, Bootsie, Dan Frey, Lauren Hanson, Justine Harkness, Allison Harm, Jack Hayes, Cinzia Iacono Pelletier, Stephanie Jolly, Ashley Kapturkiewicz, Jennifer Land, Karen Lilyquist, Edwina Lui, Heather Maigur, Maureen McMahon, Nou Moua, Alex Ricken, Christine Ricketts, Gordon Spector, Bruce Symaka, Lo'Rita Vargas, Pedro Villanueva, Dan Wittich, Jessica Yee, and many others.

TEAS® is a registered trademark of Assessment Technologies Institute (ATI), which neither sponsors nor endorses this product.

This publication is designed to provide accurate information in regard to the subject matter covered as of its publication date, with the understanding that knowledge and best practice constantly evolve. The publisher is not engaged in rendering medical, legal, accounting, or other professional service. If medical or legal advice or other expert assistance is required, the services of a competent professional should be sought. This publication is not intended for use in clinical practice or the delivery of medical care. To the fullest extent of the law, neither the Publisher nor the Editors assume any liability for any injury and/or damage to persons or property arising out of or related to any use of the material contained in this book.

© 2016 Kaplan, Inc.

Published by Kaplan Publishing, a division of Kaplan, Inc.
750 Third Avenue
New York, NY 10017

All rights reserved. The text of this publication, or any part thereof, may not be reproduced in any manner whatsoever without written permission from the publisher.

Printed in the United States of America

10 9 8 7 6 5 4 3 2 1

ISBN: 978-1-5062-1857-1

CONTENTS

FOREWORD

Congratulations! If you have picked up this book, you are considering applying to a nursing or allied health school. This is an exciting step! Your career in healthcare will provide you with many rewarding experiences and opportunities.

I speak from personal experience. Early in my career as a nurse, I was caring for a client newly diagnosed with stage 4 lung cancer. The care team had addressed his symptoms: cough, shortness of breath, fatigue, and weight loss among others. The physician had discussed the treatment plan. The social worker had offered her services. Thanks to my education, I understood the diagnosis and prognosis—the science behind the malignancy. I understood that simple remedies would not eliminate the chronic cough. I understood that the dyspnea and fatigue were inevitable and that treatment options were limited.

I also understood that no one had taken the time to *be* with the client—to sit quietly and give support, to ask questions and listen. In your role as a care provider, you will have the opportunity to offer client-centered care. You will give people respect, sensitivity, and open communication. Caring for this man during his journey did not feel like work. It was the most rewarding effort I had ever undertaken.

Because their students will someday be entrusted with the well-being of other people, healthcare programs want strong students. This only makes sense: your degree program will culminate in caring for clients who will depend on you for their health and maybe their life. We do not make or sell things. Instead, it is people and families, young and old, well and sick, who get our attention. I teach in a two-year RN program, so I fully appreciate the importance of well-prepared students. Nursing and allied healthcare programs are rigorous. I have high standards, as will your instructors. This is why school admissions can be very competitive.

To weigh the qualifications of applicants, many schools require candidates to take ATI's Test of Essential Academic Skills (TEAS®). The TEAS measures competencies in reading, math, science, and language use. Your TEAS score quantifies your academic preparedness and test-taking skills, and it is an important indicator of your potential to succeed in school.

Your nursing or allied health program will challenge you in ways that other classes have not. A lot of information will be thrown at you. You will do more academic reading than you have ever done before, and studying will require more than memorization. You must use your understanding of the knowledge of your field to recognize important facts you encounter in real-life situations and then draw sound conclusions. Especially as you move to the clinical setting, you will be making critical decisions for your clients based on information you gather.

You will also need to use math. If you want to determine the correct dose of medication for a client, you will need to be able to set up and compute proportions. You cannot trust the computer to do this—you are responsible. In any healthcare career, you are committing to lifelong learning, which means reading and evaluating research studies. Therefore, an understanding of statistics is key. Your career may take you into managing your own business or being a consultant, and then arithmetic and algebra skills will be important to you as a businessperson.

Healthcare practice requires science—anatomy and physiology, biology, and chemistry—to understand your clients' medical conditions. You may need to understand the implications of fluid balance, interpret laboratory and radiology tests, and know what effect medications can have in the body. With a good scientific education, your assessment of the client, interpretation of data, and selection of interventions will be based on evidence-based practice, not on what "feels right."

You will need strong communication skills in school and throughout your career as you speak and write to clients and colleagues. Using the correct word is critical to say what you mean to say, and you will be judged on your use of grammar. In emails and in phone conversations, your confidence and expertise must come through so people view you as someone they can depend on.

I say these things not to make you nervous and question your decision, but to emphasize the need to prepare for the TEAS. The TEAS gives you an opportunity to show schools your academic skills and ability to think like a healthcare professional. It gives you a chance to demonstrate that you are prepared for the courses ahead of you so you can gain admission to the program of your choice.

Getting into your school is just the first step toward a lifetime of opportunities. Indeed, my nursing education opened doors I didn't even imagine when I was filling out my applications. While my initial jobs were in clinical settings, I have held titles such as Nurse Manager, Clinical Reimbursement Specialist, and Subject Matter Expert. Because of my healthcare expertise and skills, I have been able to pursue consulting, business ownership, training, nursing education, and publication writing and editing. The opportunities in healthcare were so exciting and my love of learning so deep that after earning my RN, I pursued additional credentials. Today, I proudly add PhD and APRN, CNP after my name. Who knows what you will be doing in 10, 20, or 30 years? There are so many possibilities!

I encourage you to get the most that you can from this Kaplan TEAS book so that you can get into the program of your choice. Being a healthcare professional is about helping people—you will make a lasting difference in the lives of others. It is also a personally rewarding career, limited only by your imagination.

Kaplan is the premier test preparation company in the world, and we have gathered an expert team to write High-Yield Practice for the New ATI TEAS®. It is important to become comfortable with both the content and structure of the exam to ensure you obtain a TEAS score that reflects your abilities. This book will be help you succeed on this important test so this part of your application will be strong. Flip through the book. Get a sense of its content and structure. Take the full-length diagnostic test and use the Study Guide to plan your review. Use the lessons to understand how the TEAS will test certain material. Make flashcards of key terms you need to memorize. Apply your knowledge to the practice questions in the book and in the online Qbank and review the explanations. Analyze your results: What went well and what did not? Refocus your study plan based on your analysis.

Understand that pursuing a degree in nursing or an allied healthcare field is a huge commitment. Dive right in! Develop your time management skills. Seek learning opportunities. Make friends. Reach out for support. Take care of yourself. Your program is meant to be demanding—but others have come through it, and you can also. Be prepared to be successful!

Karen Lilyquist, PhD, MSN, APRN, CNP

NCLEX Instructor, Kaplan Test Prep

WELCOME TO YOUR TEAS® STUDIES!

Thank you for choosing Kaplan to help you study for the ATI TEAS®. We are honored to be part of your preparation for a career in healthcare. You will soon join the millions of nurses and other professionals who make a significant positive difference in the lives of others.

YOUR KAPLAN RESOURCES

Your Kaplan book contains:

- A full-length diagnostic test with an explanation of every question
- Tools to help you plan your studies
- Lessons that cover many of the skills and concepts on the test
  - Kaplan Methods for every question type
  - Worked examples that show the expert approach
  - Key terms in bold
  - Key takeaway summaries
  - Practice questions with explanations

Your Student Homepage offers:

- A 50-question Qbank for additional practice. The Qbank is a collection of questions you can use to create customized practice sets.

GETTING STARTED

- Go to **kaptest.com/booksonline** to register your book.
- Take the diagnostic test in Part One of this book.
- Learn, practice, and review.
- Log in to your Student Homepage at **kaptest.com** to get more practice using your Qbank.

Register Your Book

To access your Student Homepage, visit **kaptest.com/booksonline**. Choose "TEAS" from the list of tests at the top and answer the question or questions that appear.

Once you have created your username and password, you'll be able to log in to your resources at **kaptest.com**. When you're ready to use your Qbank, click **Sign In** at the upper right of the page and enter your username and password. Then click on your TEAS product to open it.

Take the Diagnostic Test

You'll find the diagnostic test in Part One of this book. Taking the diagnostic test will help you learn about the format and content of the TEAS. Your results will help you decide where to focus your studying. Set aside about 4 uninterrupted hours to take your diagnostic test. The test has four sections, and the timing for each is given in the test. You may take a 10-minute break after the second section of the test.

Also plan to set aside time to check your answers. Use the Study Planner at the end of Part One to evaluate your strengths and what areas you need to study most. Finally, begin your preparation for the TEAS by studying the explanation given for each question.

Learn, Practice, and Review

After you take the diagnostic test, you may feel confident that you can tackle most TEAS questions and only need to review a few areas or practice some skills a little more. Alternatively, you may want to study and practice much more in order to approach the test with confidence.

No matter what your performance is on the diagnostic test, you can and will improve if you set aside time to study for the TEAS. Block out study time on your calendar, just as you would write down any other appointment. These blocks of time are appointments with yourself, so keep them!

A great deal of research shows that we learn better in shorter, more frequent study sessions. Therefore, plan to study at least three days a week for one to three hours, rather than one or two days a week for four or more hours.

Also, consider how much time you have between now and when you will take the TEAS. Estimate how many hours you need to study to master the material. Divide the number of hours of study by the number of weeks. This is the number of hours you need to study each week. Then divide that number by the number of days you will study each week. This is the number of hours per day you need to study. Here's an example:

Taking the TEAS in 4 weeks, need to study about 40 hours, and can study 4 days a week

Calculate hours per week:
40 hours ÷ 4 weeks = 10 hours/week

Calculate hours per day:
10 hours/week ÷ 4 days/week = 2.5 hours/day

This person will block out 2.5 hours on 4 days each week for the next 4 weeks to prepare for the TEAS.

Finally, every time you sit down to study, set a goal for that session. Examples of goals are "Complete two Reading lessons and understand the explanation of every practice question," or "Memorize the path of blood through the body and be able to diagram it." Setting a goal at the beginning of your study session sets you up to feel great when you have achieved it at the end of the session.

Use Your Online Resources

The Qbank in your Student Homepage allows you to get focused practice in particular content areas. A great way to use this resource is to create a practice set of five questions in one topic, try your best on them, and then review the explanations thoroughly. If you missed a question, review the explanation until you understand the correct answer. Then do the question again. Of course, you already know the answer. However, actually doing the question correctly will reinforce the memory in your brain, helping you to retain the knowledge so you will know it on Test Day.

Want More?

This Kaplan book and the Qbank on your Student Homepage will give you an excellent foundation for your TEAS studies. For over 500 additional practice questions, look for Kaplan's *ATI TEAS® Qbank* coming November 2016. For even more comprehensive instruction in TEAS topics and a second, online full-length test, look for *ATI TEAS® Strategies, Practice, & Review with 2 Practice Tests* coming January 2017.

MANAGING STRESS

You have a lot riding on the TEAS. However, you're also doing the work you need to do to reach your goals. Unfortunately, sometimes just knowing that you're working hard won't make your test anxiety go away. Thus, here are some stress management tips from our long experience of helping students prepare for standardized tests.

Clock in and out: Once you've set up a study schedule for yourself, treat it like a job. That is, imagine clocking yourself in and out of TEAS studies according to that schedule. Do your best to stick to your schedule, and when you're not "clocked in," don't let yourself think about the TEAS. That will help you release your stress about the test in between study sessions.

Don't punish yourself: If you get tired or overwhelmed or discouraged when studying, don't respond by pushing yourself harder. Instead, step away and engage in a relaxing activity like going for a walk, watching a movie, or playing with your cat or dog. Then, when you're ready, return to your studies with fresh eyes.

Breathe: Remember to take deep breaths, consciously using your diaphragm to breathe "into your stomach." This breathing technique will help your muscles to relax, and when your body relaxes, your mind relaxes as well.

Set small, manageable goals: Each week, set manageable goals for your TEAS progress. Then reward yourself when you've achieved them. Examples of small goals might be:

- This week, memorize and practice the Kaplan Method for Science until I no longer have to think about what the steps of the Method are.
- This week, do 20 math questions and practice each until I can move confidently and efficiently from the information provided to the correct answer.
- This week, review all the spelling rules that the TEAS is likely to test until I can identify words that use them and words that are common exceptions.

Keep yourself healthy: Good health, adequate rest, and regular interactions with friends and family make it easier to cope with the challenges of studying. Stay on a regular sleep schedule as much as possible during your studies, eat well, continue to exercise, and spend time with those you care about and those who help you feel good about yourself. Also, don't fuel your studies with caffeine and sugar. Those substances may make you feel alert, but they can also damage focus.

Remind yourself why you are doing this: If you feel tempted to pass up a planned study session because you're tired or something comes up that feels like a higher priority, remind yourself how important a good score on the TEAS is. Success on this test will open the doors to an important educational credential and many career opportunities after that. If you planned to study for 90 minutes and don't think you can study for that long, then study for 30 minutes. You will make progress toward the score you want, and you will feel better about yourself than if you "blow it off." You may even be surprised at how fast the 30 minutes go by and decide that you can study longer after all.

Keep the right mindset: Most importantly, keep telling yourself that you *can* do this. Don't fall into the trap of thinking that you're not "allowed" to feel confident yet. That's a self-punishing attitude that will only hurt you. Rather, remember that confidence breeds success. So let yourself be confident about your abilities. You're obviously ambitious and intelligent, so walk into the TEAS knowing that about yourself.

If you get discouraged, make a list: If you start to wonder if you'll ever reach your TEAS goals, stop what you're doing and make a list of everything you're good at. List *every specific skill* that you are bringing to the TEAS. Here are some examples:

- Finding the main point of a passage
- Using suffixes to tell whether a word is a noun, verb, or adjective
- Identifying what a math question is asking for
- Comparing two fractions to find which one is larger
- Naming the organ systems of the human body
- Explaining how oxygen reaches tissues in the body

Post that list of things you're good at somewhere you'll see it every day and add to it as you continue to study. It will be a long list in no time! We at Kaplan recommend making this list because many people focus too heavily on their weaknesses while preparing for a standardized test. But if you only focus on your weaknesses, you aren't seeing an objective picture. There *are* TEAS skills you're good at. Keep that in mind and focus on building on those strengths.

ALSO IMPORTANT . . .

- Think about what school(s) you will apply to. What are your criteria for a program? Consider the degrees offered, geographic location, cost, campus culture, and other factors.
- Research the colleges and universities that offer the kind of program you're interested in. Visit their websites to learn more about the admissions process and talk to an admissions officer about the school's acceptance criteria for prospective students.
- Talk to alumni of your target programs to learn about how their education has prepared them for their careers and what surprises and challenges they have encountered.

By researching the school(s) you'll apply to, you will be able to choose a school that is a good fit for you and your goals. You'll experience much less stress as you work toward your degree than you would if you are not in a school that meets your needs.

THE ROAD TO TEST DAY

You've read this book. You know what to expect on the TEAS. You've studied a lot. Your Test Day is approaching. How can you make sure you do your best?

The Week Before Test Day

Rest: Make sure you're on a regular sleep schedule.

Rehearse: Find out where you will be taking the test and consider doing a "dry run." Drive or commute to the test site around the same time of day as your test will be. You don't want to be surprised by traffic or road construction on Test Day. You also don't want to get delayed or stressed out trying to figure out where to park, which way to go after you get off the bus, or where the restrooms are.

Review: Do a high-level review. Flip through the lessons and rework a few practice problems here and there to reinforce all of the good habits you've developed in your preparation. (Redoing practice problems you've already done is fine: you can actually learn a lot that way about how to approach those types of questions more efficiently in the future.)

Stop: Two days before the test, stop studying—no studying at all! You're not likely to learn anything new in those two days, and you'll get a lot more out of walking into the test feeling rested.

Relax: The evening before the test, do something fun (but not crazy or tiring). Maybe you could have a nice dinner (without alcohol), watch a movie, catch up on housework (a clean house is relaxing for some people), or play a game.

Go to bed: Go to bed early enough to get a full night's sleep (7–8 hours) before the day of the exam.

On Test Day Itself

Warm up: Before you take the test, do a TEAS warm-up. This will help your brain get ready to function at its best. Don't take any practice materials into the testing center, but do a few easy practice questions at home or work before you leave for the test.

Don't let nerves derail you: You have every reason to feel confident. You have prepared for this test! But if you do find yourself getting nervous or losing focus, sit back in your seat and place your feet flat on the floor. Then take a few deep breaths and close your eyes or focus them on something other than the computer screen or test booklet for a moment. Remind yourself that you have studied diligently and are ready for the TEAS. When you're ready, reengage with the test.

Keep moving: Don't let yourself get bogged down on any one question. You can come back to questions that you aren't sure about, so skip questions whenever they threaten to slow you down or to steal time from the other questions. There is no penalty for a wrong answer on the TEAS, so make sure to answer every question before time is called, even if you have to guess on some questions. Also, remember to use the multiple-choice format to your advantage: if you can eliminate one or two answer choices as incorrect, you have greatly increased your chances of guessing correctly.

Don't assess yourself: This is very important. As you're testing, don't let yourself stop and think about how you *feel* you're doing. Taking a standardized test hardly ever *feels* good. Your own impressions of how it's going are totally unreliable. So, instead of focusing on that, remind yourself that you're prepared and that you are going to succeed, even if you feel discouraged as the test is underway.

After the test, celebrate! You've prepared, practiced, and performed like a champion. Now that the test is over, it's time to congratulate yourself on a job well done. Celebrate responsibly with friends and family and enjoy the rest of your day, knowing you just took an important step toward reaching your goals.

GOOD LUCK!

We at Kaplan wish you the very best in your studies, on the TEAS, and in your career as a healthcare professional. If you have feedback or questions about this book, please email us at TEASfeedback@kaplan.com

ABOUT THE TEAS

WHAT IS THE TEAS?

The ATI TEAS was developed to evaluate the academic readiness of applicants to health science programs, such as nursing programs. *TEAS* stands for Test of Essential Academic Skills. *ATI* is the name of the testmaker and stands for Assessment Technologies Institute.

More programs accept TEAS scores than any other health science admissions test, but some programs want applicants to submit scores from other tests. Therefore, before studying for the TEAS and taking the test, check with the schools you're interested in to make sure they accept a TEAS score.

What Does the TEAS Test?

The questions you will see on the TEAS assess knowledge and skills that have been identified by health science schools as relevant to assessing your readiness to begin a college program of study. The material tested is typically taught in grades 7–12. The TEAS tests material in four content areas as follows:

Content Area	Number of Questions (Number of Scored Questions)	Time Limit
Reading	53 (47)	64 minutes
Mathematics	36 (32)	54 minutes
Break		10 minutes
Science	53 (47)	63 minutes
English and language usage	28 (24)	28 minutes
Total	**170 (150)**	**219 minutes**

The 20 unscored questions are experimental questions included to test their validity. You will not know whether a question is scored or unscored, so do your best on every question.

There is no penalty for wrong answers on the TEAS, so make sure to answer every question. Even if you need to guess, you might get the question right. If you can eliminate one or two answer choices as clearly incorrect, then you increase your chances of guessing correctly.

This book is organized to correspond to the content areas of the test. Part One contains a diagnostic test and answers and explanations for every question on the test, as well as a Study Guide to help you use your test results. After that are the following sections:

- Part Two: Reading
- Part Three: Mathematics
- Part Four: Science
- Part Five: English and Language Usage

Part Six provides answers and explanations for every practice question you find at the end of each lesson in Parts Two through Five.

How Is the ATI TEAS Different From the TEAS V?

The retirement date for the TEAS V is August 31, 2016. After this date, prospective health science students will take the ATI TEAS. There are three key differences between the old and new editions of the test:

- A calculator is now permitted on the *Mathematics* section. If you are taking the test on a computer, a four-function calculator is embedded in the onscreen test interface. If you are taking the pencil-and-paper version of the test, the proctor will give you a four-function calculator. You may not bring your own calculator to the test.
- The four content areas of the test have not changed. However, the specific competencies emphasized in each have been realigned in response to the feedback of educators about the skills that entry-level health science students should possess.
- The previous test reported all scores as a percentage. The ATI TEAS reports your composite score as a number and continues to report your content area scores as percentages.

TEAS LOGISTICS

Learning all you can about the TEAS will help you have a smooth experience on Test Day, and you'll be able to submit your applications to schools efficiently. Just as preparing for the questions you will see on the test is important, so too is preparing to register and take the test.

How to Register for the Test

Be sure to register early because seating for each test administration is limited. One way to register for the TEAS is to go to the testmaker's website at **atitesting.com**. You will need to create an account and be logged in to the site to register for the test. Click on the Online Store and select Register for... TEAS. You will be asked where you want to take the test. Then you will be asked for billing information. The fee for the test if you register through the ATI website is $56. You can also contact ATI at 800-667-7531 to register for the test. Business hours are Monday to Friday, 7:00 AM to 7:00 PM Central Time.

Another way to register is to contact the school to which you plan to apply and ask for a list of TEAS testing locations. Many nursing and allied health programs administer the TEAS on campus, and registration for the test is sometimes available through the school.

If you register for the test through ATI, your registration is final. To change your test date, you will need to register again and pay the test fee again. If you registered for the test through a school and want to change your test date, contact the school to find out what the policy is.

When you register for the TEAS, you can request that the school at which you are taking your test receive your score at no additional cost. If you want to submit your score to other schools, go to the testmaker's website at **atitesting.com** and use the Online Store to order your transcript(s). The fee is $27 per transcript.

If you want to request accommodations for a disability, contact ATI at 800-667-7531.

Test Administration

On the day of your test, arrive at least 15 minutes early so the proctor can verify your identity and get you checked in. Proctors will monitor you throughout the test, and they will intervene if they observe disruptive behavior.

Bring the following items to the testing site:

- Government-issued identification with a current photograph, your signature, and your permanent address. Examples include a driver's license or state ID card, military ID, US passport, or US permanent resident card (green card).
  - Not acceptable: Student ID card, credit card
- Two sharpened No. 2 pencils with attached erasers
  - Not acceptable: Pens, highlighters, mechanical pencils, separate erasers
- Your ATI assessment ID. You receive this in a confirmation email when you register for the test.
- If your test will be online, you will need to know your ATI account username and password so you can log in.

Your testing site may issue specific instructions about Test Day. Read the instructions carefully and follow them so you are not denied admittance when you show up to take your test.

Do *not* bring these items to the test:

- Electronic or Internet-enabled devices of any kind. These include cell or smart phones, portable music players, tablets, and digital or smart watches. Leave these in your car or at home. Do not bring a calculator—one will be provided to you.
- Clothing and accessories such as a jacket, hat, or sunglasses. The proctor may inspect any article of clothing.
  - Exception: The proctors have discretion to permit items of religious apparel to be worn.
- Other personal items such as a purse, backpack, or bag of any kind
- Food and beverages
  - Exception: Items documented as medically necessary

The following items will be provided to you by the proctor:

- A four-function calculator, if you are taking the paper-and-pencil version of the test. If your test is on the computer, then the calculator will be onscreen.
- Scratch paper. You may not write on this paper before the test begins or during your break, and you must return all scratch paper to the proctor at the end of the test.

Note that during the test, if you need to leave for any reason, you must raise your hand and be excused by the proctor. While you are out of the room, the timer will continue to count down; any time you miss cannot be made up. If you need the proctor's assistance for any other reason, such as a technical malfunction with your computer, raise your hand. Finally, if you find the test setting uncomfortable or inadequate, report your concern to the proctor before leaving the room at the end of the test.

Your Scores

You will receive a composite score reflecting your overall performance and a sub-score for each content area. If you take the test online, you will see your scores immediately upon completion of the test. If you take the paper-and-pencil version, your scores will show up in your ATI online account within 48 hours of ATI's receiving the test from the testing site. In addition to your scores, the report will identify topics on which you missed questions. You can access your score report at the testmaker's website at any time by logging in.

Some schools require a certain composite score for admission, while others require you to meet a minimum score in each content area. Some schools do not have any specific cutoff scores for admission. Be sure to check with the program(s) to which you are applying to find out the requirements.

Be aware that some schools with a cutoff score require applicants to achieve the minimum score within a certain number of test administrations. For example, a school may require applicants to obtain the minimum score by taking the TEAS no more than twice. In this case, if you did not achieve the cutoff score after taking the test twice but did get a score above the threshold the third time you took the test, your application would still not meet that school's criteria for admission.

Finally, just because a school gives a minimum score or scores for admission, that does not mean that every applicant who meets or exceeds that score(s) is accepted. Other aspects of your application are generally considered as well. In the same way, a school that does not have a minimum TEAS score may nonetheless mostly accept students with high scores. Again, research the schools to which you are applying to find out what they seek in a successful candidate.

Note: All information in this section "About the TEAS" is current as this book goes to press. Check the ATI website at **atitesting.com** for the most up-to-date information.

TEAS Diagnostic Test

This diagnostic test is designed to help guide you in your preparation for the TEAS. You will learn several things from taking this test.

What's on the TEAS?

The test you are about to take is designed to be very similar to the TEAS. This test is the same length as the TEAS. The questions are in the same multiple-choice format, and the knowledge and skills tested reflect those you will need to do well on Test Day. By the end of this test, you will have a very good idea of what to expect on Test Day in each of the four content areas tested: *Reading*, *Mathematics*, *Science*, and *English language and usage*.

Furthermore, following the diagnostic test are comprehensive answers and explanations of every question. Read all the explanations—of the questions you got right as well as those you got wrong. When you got a question correct, the explanation will validate and reinforce your approach, or it might reveal a strategy that would have gotten you to the right answer more quickly and confidently. When you missed a question, the explanation will teach you what you need to know to get a similar question right on Test Day.

What Is It Like to Take the TEAS?

The TEAS is a 3.5-hour test. It's a long test! To evaluate your current mental endurance, take this diagnostic test under test-like conditions. Set aside a block of 4 hours when you won't be interrupted and find a quiet space. You won't be allowed to eat or drink during the test, so reserve refreshments for your breaks. Shut down email, social media, and other distractions.

If you find that fatigue interferes with your ability to do your best toward the end of the test, then plan to build up your mental endurance gradually, studying for longer and longer periods of time until you can focus on test material for several hours.

What Are My Strengths? Where Are My Opportunities?

After you take this diagnostic test, use the Answers and Explanations immediately following the test to check your answers. Then use the Study Planner charts to analyze what content and skills you already feel comfortable with and which areas you need to study more. Use this analysis to plan where you will focus your study time.

Reading

Directions You have 64 minutes to answer 53 questions. Do not work on any other section of the test during this time.

Questions 1–2 are based on the following passage.

The first detective stories, written by Edgar Allan Poe and Arthur Conan Doyle, emerged in the mid-nineteenth century, at a time when there was enormous public interest in science. The newspapers of the day continually publicized the latest scientific discoveries, and scientists were acclaimed as the heroes of the age. Poe and Conan Doyle shared this fascination with the methodical, logical approach used by scientists in their experiments and instilled their detective heroes with outstanding powers of scientific reasoning.

Granted, public knowledge and attitudes about science at the time were not the same as today's, and Doyle's lifelong interest in ghost hunting might appear malapropos for a rationalist. These apparent quirks aside, the spirit of science is hardly better exemplified or better known than in Doyle's stories, especially in the methods and attitude of his fictional detective, Sherlock Holmes.

1. According to the passage, Poe and Conan Doyle were similar in that

   (A) they both enjoyed gothic horror.
   (B) they wrote about heroes whose rational approach mirrored that of real-life scientists.
   (C) they wrote true accounts of police detective work for newspapers.
   (D) they were scientists.

2. The word "malapropos" means that an object or behavior is

   (A) scientific.
   (B) appropriate.
   (C) endearingly quirky.
   (D) out of place.

J. R. Sorensen, a critic of the judicial system, wrote, "In each of the last three years, a court in this country has awarded a settlement in excess of $300 million. This is a travesty of justice, and it unfairly burdens the court system, setting precedent as well as incentive for more and more suits of this kind."

3. What would Sorensen likely suggest to alleviate the strain on the courts?

   (A) There should be fewer lawsuits.
   (B) Courts should stop awarding such excessive settlements.
   (C) Lawsuits should name more than one defendant.
   (D) Larger out-of-court settlements should be awarded to ensure they meet victims' needs.

For do-it-yourself types, the cost of getting regular oil changes seems unnecessary. After all, the steps are fairly easy as long as you exercise basic safety precautions. First, make sure that the car is stationary and on a level surface. Always use the emergency brake to ensure that the car does not roll on top of you. Next, locate the drain plug for the oil under the engine. Remember to place the oil drain pan under the plug before you start. When the oil is drained fully, wipe off the drain plug and the plug opening and then replace the drain plug. Next, simply place your funnel in the engine and pour in new oil. Be sure to return the oil cap when you are done. Finally, run the engine for a minute and then check the dipstick to see if you need more oil in your engine.

4. After draining the old oil from the engine, you should

   (A) replace the oil cap.
   (B) run the engine for a moment and check the dipstick.
   (C) wipe off and replace the drain plug.
   (D) engage the emergency brake.

Questions 5–10 are based on the following passage.

Does true happiness come from within or from without? Do we achieve fulfillment when life circumstances happen to satisfy our desires, as the modern utilitarian view maintains? Or, on the contrary, is it as the ancient Stoics and Buddhists claim, that we become happy only through renouncing material wants and cultivating a positive perception and attitude?

In his landmark work, *The Happiness Hypothesis*, psychologist Jonathan Haidt shows that the source of happiness is neither internal nor external—or, more accurately, that it is both. Having embarked upon an ambitious project of cataloging the world's wisdom and then looking for scientific results that verify ancient proverbs, Haidt establishes that true happiness comes from "between," requiring a mix of internal and external conditions. Some of those conditions are within you, like your perspective and personality. Other conditions are external. Just as plants need sun, water, and good soil to thrive, people need love, work, and a connection to something larger to be happy.

5. The main idea of the passage is that

  (A) Buddhism and utilitarianism both fail to explain or create happiness.

  (B) ancient proverbs and philosophies contain wisdom that science has only recently acknowledged.

  (C) even if a person has the best attitude in the world, there will be a limit to his or her emotional endurance.

  (D) happiness requires a combination of the right internal attitude as well as external life circumstances.

6. Which belief system states that people's happiness comes from the state of the world?

  (A) Utilitarianism

  (B) Experimental psychology

  (C) Buddhism

  (D) Stoicism

7. Why did the author of the passage describe utilitarianism in the second sentence?

  (A) To support the main purpose of the passage by explaining the utilitarian perspective on happiness

  (B) To provide an example of how a person can experience happiness from "between"

  (C) To offer evidence against the idea that happiness is under internal control

  (D) To provide an example of a belief system in which happiness is held to be influenced by external factors

8. What is the author's main goal in writing this passage?

  (A) To argue that both internal attitude and life circumstances play a role in a person's happiness

  (B) To explain that there are many views on how to achieve happiness, dating back thousands of years

  (C) To argue that, while psychologists like Jonathon Haidt think they have figured out happiness, achieving happiness is not as simple as they claim

  (D) To compare and contrast ancient Buddhist and Stoic beliefs on the topic of happiness

9. Suppose a new study revealed that the happiest people tend to have few attachments to material objects and want little besides what they already possess. What effect would this evidence have if the author included it in the passage?

  (A) It would weaken the claim that happiness comes from "within."

  (B) It would challenge the claim that happiness comes from "without."

  (C) It would strengthen the claim that happiness comes from "without."

  (D) It would support the claim that happiness comes from "between."

10. With which of the following statements would the author of the passage most likely NOT agree?

  (A) Social services that provide food and housing to refugees and foster their sense of belonging make the world a happier place.

  (B) Because there is more than one way to be happy, even someone in difficult circumstances can find joy with the right outlook.

  (C) People who appreciate what they have tend to be happier than those who always seek to complain.

  (D) Even a person who has everything can be unhappy, and their loved ones may not be able to help.

11. Start with the figure below. Follow the instructions to rearrange its parts.

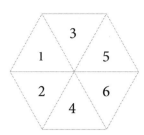

1. Switch the positions of numbers 1 and 6.
2. Switch the positions of numbers 2 and 5.
3. Switch the positions of numbers 4 and 5.

The shape now looks like which of the following?

(A)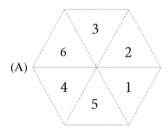

(B)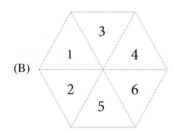

(C)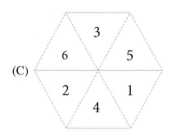

(D)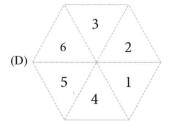

Many people strongly dislike snakes, finding them unappealing to look at and uncomfortable to touch. On the contrary, snakes are fascinating creatures, with their iridescent scales and elegant movements.

12. Which word best describes the author's attitude toward snakes?

(A) Disgusted
(B) Appreciative
(C) Uninterested
(D) Fearful

Dear Grandma,

Thanks so much for the birthday card! I love it. The flowers are so pretty. It's just like your garden. When the snow melts here in the Rockies, I'll come visit you and we can plant flowers together.

I love you!

13. Based on the information in this letter, the writer's birthday is most likely in

(A) January.
(B) May.
(C) August.
(D) September.

"Akira Kurosawa," a paper by Jack Schroeder for English 410 (first draft)

The Japanese filmmaker Akira Kurosawa (1910–1988) is renowned as one of the greatest directors in film history. He directed thirty films in his almost sixty-year career, and among his movies are classics like *Rashomon, Seven Samurai,* and *Yojimbo*. His first feature work was an action movie, but he later turned to William Shakespeare for inspiration, freely adapting the Bard's plays for his own films: *Throne of Blood* (*Macbeth*), *The Bad Sleep Well* (*Hamlet*), and *Ran* (*King Lear*). His films are highly regarded for their epic scope, striking visuals, and Kurosawa's keen interest in every aspect of filmmaking, including scriptwriting, casting, editing, and even set design. In 1990, he accepted a Lifetime Achievement from the Academy of Motion Picture Arts and Sciences…

English 410: Advanced Topics in Shakespeare Adaptation

This seminar will examine the influence of Shakespeare's plays and poetry on works in other media, including fiction, cinema, music, and the visual arts. Students will be expected to conduct independent research into adaptations of Shakespeare's work and bring their findings to class.

STUDENT SURVEY! FREE MOVIE NIGHT!

The University Student Association has received funding for extracurricular activities. We have decided to organize a weekly film night but want to hear from you! What kind of films would you like to see in our new series? Please email us your suggestions for movies we should include. Hope to hear from you!

____ Silent Comedies

____ Hollywood Horror

____ Classic International Japanese and German Cinema

____ English Spy Movies

14. Jack Schroeder is very concerned about getting high grades. Given the paper he is currently writing for English 410, which of the following is he most likely to do in response to the student survey?

 (A) State his preference for Hollywood Horror because he wants to see *Throne of Blood*.
 (B) Contact the Student Association and name some movies by Akira Kurosawa the Association should show.
 (C) Choose English Spy Movies because he hopes there's still room in a very popular course on the spy novels of Ian Fleming and John le Carré.
 (D) Ignore the petition because he will be too busy reading Shakespeare plays to watch movies.

Questions 15–16 are based on the following story.

For red-blooded American boys, baseball is a rite of passage. It's something passed on from father to son that creates a bond both between and within generations of men. Toby knew this because his father had explained it to him. Today's game was the final game of the season, but it was also the final league game, period, for this young man. Soon after his 16th birthday, he would be headed to the military academy as a fresh cadet, and his time for recreational sports would be finished.

As the sky cleared and sun at last rushed into the room, Toby smiled, knowing that the game would proceed as scheduled. It had to, if only because his father would be there and it would be the last opportunity he would have to see Toby play. Now the birds began to appear here and there. Toby had a special feeling about today. He got out his baseball glove and waited for his dad to arrive to take him to the game.

15. What were the author's intentions in writing this passage?

 (A) To tell a story about a significant life milestone
 (B) To inform the reader about the cultural and historical significance of baseball
 (C) To argue for the importance of rituals in moving into new stages of life
 (D) To share an opinion about baseball's cultural relevance

16. The mood of the character in the passage is

 (A) sad.
 (B) careless.
 (C) uneasy.
 (D) eager.

Questions 17–18 are based on the following statements.

The school board is considering the amount of homework students should be assigned and has solicited input from parents. The following statements were submitted to the board.

More Homework!

Don't get me wrong. I don't exactly have fond memories of spending my evenings struggling through my high school chemistry work, but did I learn the subject better by putting the time in? You bet I did. And I didn't become a chemist, but as a small-business owner putting in those late nights when I just have to get my books up-to-date, or make the work schedule, or just clean up after a particularly busy day, I'm thankful that my parents didn't let me shirk my duties way back when. Being self-employed means no one's going to stand there and make you get your work done, so you better have the wherewithal to do what needs to be done without someone on your back. You learn this by challenging yourself and doing the work you signed up for.

We're Really Starting Young with the Life Sentences Now

We're turning ourselves into a society with no boundaries and no work-life balance (the very fact that we have a term to describe this concept tells you that it's no longer a given), and we're starting younger and younger. My third-grade daughter is sitting at the kitchen table with me until nine o'clock at night trying to get her social studies homework done. Why? What happens if she's limited to the 36 hours per week she spends with her teacher? Will she know not quite enough about Jamestown to ever be successful in life? Is this what we're trading our quality time for each night? I don't want my kid to get an ulcer before she's even out of grade school, just to prepare her for the theoretical point in life when this ridiculous amount of work might actually become necessary rather than contrived.

17. What do the two authors disagree about?

   (A) They disagree over whether career success is important in life.
   (B) They disagree over how heavy the student workload actually is.
   (C) They disagree over whether the benefit of completing homework is worth the effort.
   (D) They disagree over whether quality time with one's family is worthwhile.

18. Which of the following statements, if true, would weaken both arguments in this passage?

   (A) A study shows that students who took heavier course loads and participated in more academic extracurricular activities showed a decreased ability to work independently in their later careers.
   (B) A survey of students in kindergarten through grade 12 found that most considered their academic load to be minimal and unchallenging.
   (C) In a state-wide survey, young children consistently listed "learning together" as one of the most enjoyable and important things they did with their parents.
   (D) A comparative study of syllabi shows that, on average, the academic workload at the college level has remained stable.

The English language is an amalgam of several other languages, but relies most heavily on Latin. Over time, new English words have often been created from Latin prefixes and roots. Thus, the word *ambidextrous* combines the Latin root *ambi*, meaning "both," and *dexter*, meaning "right-handed." Literally, this means "right-handed on both sides," but we interpret it as meaning being capable of using both hands equally well.

19. The word "ambidextrous" is used in the paragraph in order to

   (A) provide a supporting detail for the main idea.
   (B) introduce the primary topic.
   (C) illustrate a word that is always interpreted literally.
   (D) give an example of a Latin word.

Dear Janelle,

Sorry for taking so long to get back to you but it's so busy this time of year, as you know. To answer your question, the Marketing Department has decided to implement the new direct marketing campaign via social media because we feel that social media users tend to be the demographic—younger, cosmopolitan, educated—that our new app is designed to serve. It's an exciting opportunity for our group as a whole. The decision has already been made, but I thank you for your input.

Best,
Asafa

20. What is the author's purpose in writing this memo?

   (A) She is explaining the basis for a marketing decision.
   (B) She is ignoring Janelle's input.
   (C) She is apologizing for an unfortunate outcome.
   (D) She is suggesting that Janelle make more use of social media.

Questions 21–23 are based on the following passage.

The history of astronomy is very much the history of what became visible to human beings and when. The four brightest moons of Jupiter were the first objects in the solar system discovered with the use of the telescope. Their discovery played a central role in Galileo's famous argument in support of the Copernican model of the solar system, in which the planets are described as revolving around the sun. For several hundred years, scientific understanding of these moons was slow to develop. But spectacular close-up photographs sent back by the 1979 *Voyager* missions forever changed our perception of these moons, as did improved observations from the powerful Hubble Space Telescope.

Of course, there's a reason these moons were the first to be discovered—after Earth's own moon, of course. The table below shows the brightness (apparent magnitude) of different solar system objects as seen from Earth. There are nearer planetary satellites; indeed, Mars has two moons. However, distance is only one variable affecting brightness. Size is also very important. Note that on this scale, the higher the number, the fainter the object appears.

Name of Moon (Planet It Orbits)	Apparent Magnitude
Luna (Earth's moon)	−12.6
Ganymede (Jupiter)	4.8
Calipso (Jupiter)	5.6
Phobos (Mars)	11.3
Charon (Pluto)	15.6

21. The main idea of the passage is that

(A) the four moons of Jupiter provided strong evidence of Copernicus's solar system model.
(B) the four moons of Jupiter provided strong evidence of Galileo's solar system model.
(C) The telescope completely changed our understanding of the universe.
(D) astronomy has advanced based on our ability to perceive different celestial objects.

22. Given the information in the passage, it's reasonable to assume that

(A) the four moons of Jupiter would be brighter than Earth's moon if they were closer.
(B) the planets were all discovered before their moons because the planets are larger.
(C) the more powerful the telescope, the fainter the objects it can be used to discover.
(D) an astronomer can use an object's brightness to determine how far away it is.

23. Based on the passage, which is the most reasonable value for the apparent magnitude of the sun?

(A) −26.7
(B) −5.4
(C) 6.9
(D) 31.2

Chef Marion: "You should add salt to water you wish to boil. Because salty water has a higher boiling point than unsalted water, you can cook at a higher temperature with it. Also, some foods, like pasta, taste better when cooked in salted water."

24. Which of the following is an opinion Chef Marion offers?

(A) Food is healthier when cooked in unsalted water.
(B) Added salt raises the temperature of boiling water.
(C) Some foods taste better when cooked in salted water.
(D) Salted water enables food to be cooked more quickly.

When painting a room, initially decide on the general color desired, for example, some shade of blue. Buy a small amount of several blue shades to test out at home. Paint a small patch of wall with each color. After letting the paint dry, determine which blue you prefer, buy an adequate amount of that color, and paint the entire room.

25. Which of the following is NOT a step in painting a room?

(A) Painting small areas with blue and other colors
(B) Choosing colors from dry samples
(C) Deciding on the general color for the room
(D) Buying small amounts of paint

Questions 26–27 are based on the following passage.

The English-born fashion designer Charles Frederick Worth is widely considered the inventor of haute couture, establishing new benchmarks for quality of construction and luxuriousness of materials. At his Paris salon, he created grand clothes for European royalty, including the Empress Eugénie. Despite his illustrious clientele and painstaking craftsmanship, his clothing was also suitable for everyday life. Yet, his importance goes beyond making beautiful dresses. Because of his relentless self-promotion—by the 1870s, his name was familiar not only to the wealthy women who could afford his creations but also to the readers of the newly popular women's magazines—he was the forerunner of today's superstar fashion designers. Thus, the structure of the fashion industry today owes a great deal to this nineteenth-century entrepreneur.

26. According to the passage, which of the following contributes to a piece of clothing being considered haute couture?

   (A) Its suitability for everyday life
   (B) Its appeal to European royalty
   (C) Its quality of construction and luxuriousness of materials
   (D) Its creator's relentless self-promotion

27. Which of the following statements, if true, would strengthen the author's argument?

   (A) Worth has a prominent entry in an encyclopedia of fashion throughout history.
   (B) Many fashion designers today seek to be well-known among people who cannot afford their clothes.
   (C) Worth's clothes for the Empress Eugénie are still considered a model for designers who receive commissions from European royal families.
   (D) Worth was not only famous during his lifetime but ran a highly profitable business.

What a week it had been! When Jason arrived late to work on Friday, he told his boss there had been a big accident on Maple Street and the police had shut down all the lanes. There was a detour, but unfortunately larger trucks could not take that route and had to backtrack several blocks instead. When Jason had finally arrived in the parking lot at work, he could only find spaces for compact cars. Jason's boss accepted the explanation, this time. At least Jason could sleep in the next morning.

28. Which of the following was NOT implied by Jason's story?

   (A) Jason had been late to work earlier in the week.
   (B) Jason drove down Maple on his way in to work.
   (C) Jason drives a larger truck.
   (D) Jason had to backtrack several blocks.

The Most Excellent Order of the British Empire, or MBE, is the order of chivalry of the British constitutional monarchy. In 1917, King George V identified a need to fill a gap in the British honors system, specifically to recognize those who had served in noncombat roles in the Great War (what would come to be known as the First World War). The war had lasted much longer than expected, and there was no way to acknowledge the contributions that civilians had made to the war effort at home or that military personnel had made in support positions. Soon after its foundation, the order was divided into military and civil divisions, and these days it continues to fulfill its original purpose in new ways, rewarding people for their contributions to public service, the arts and science, sports, and charity and welfare organizations.

29. Which of the following identifies the structure of the passage?

   (A) Biographical narrative
   (B) Compare and contrast
   (C) Opinion and rationale
   (D) Problem and solution

Total national expenditures on healthcare exceed those on transportation and related infrastructure, the justice system (including law enforcement), and even agriculture and food distribution. Could healthcare cost less than it does? Some people argue that high costs are inevitable because doctors have student loans to pay and pharmaceutical companies have a responsibility to their shareholders. However, it is worth looking at the largest costs to see whether a savings of a few percent might be possible. Considering the cost breakdown below, not much savings could be found in, for example, syringes, cotton swabs, and other disposable (nondurable) medical products. On the other hand, reducing the top two or three categories by a few percentage points could have a significant impact.

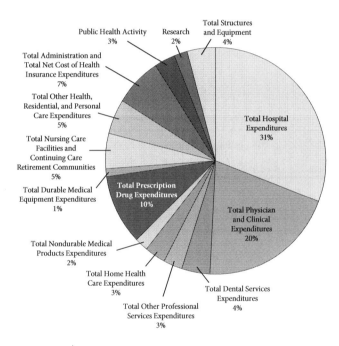

30. Which of the following cost-saving measures would the author of the passage be least likely to support?

(A) A pooling of hospitals' and clinics' procurement of surgical tools, such as laser scalpels, so these instruments are purchased at lower cost
(B) A self-service medical portal that lowers the incidence of unnecessary hospital and physician visits
(C) Incentives to encourage pharmaceutical companies to make the most commonly prescribed drugs available as less expensive generics
(D) A more efficient system of rural hospitals that would reduce the number of buildings and amount spent on overhead.

Dear Editor,

Last week, this newspaper reported on the mayor's misguided plan to open two new municipally sponsored daycare centers. The mayor cites a lack of affordable child care as the reason that many parents, predominantly mothers, are not able to return to work. He promises that the daycare centers would improve the economy by providing high-paying jobs for daycare workers while also allowing skilled workers to return to work. Does he not realize that the average hourly wage in this county is barely $16, with many citizens earning much less, while he is promising daycare workers $14? Why should mothers go back to work for a net gain of $2 an hour, while other people raise their children? One parent, not necessarily a female parent, should stay at home to raise children until they're old enough to go to school. This is a goal worth investing in.

31. What is the flaw in the main argument of this letter to the editor?

(A) The $2 net gain calculation assumes equal hours for the parent and daycare worker.
(B) It assumes that one daycare worker will be required for each parent who wants to return to work.
(C) The mayor assumes that all parents are skilled workers.
(D) The author clearly has a personal opinion about whether parents should stay home with their children.

Jim was always smiling, so his friends complimented him on his sunny disposition.

32. Which of the following would be the best word to substitute for "sunny"?

(A) Rude
(B) Pleasant
(C) Grave
(D) Wooden

Thomas: "Our study group should concentrate on the respiratory system because that area of study made up a major portion of last year's anatomy and physiology final."

Martina: "Should we really waste valuable time on the respiratory system? Everyone knows our professor is new to the faculty and is an expert in the cardiovascular system."

33. Which word best describes Martina's tone?

(A) Challenging
(B) Encouraging
(C) Understanding
(D) Puzzled

Questions 34–38 are based on the following passage.

In the young American democracy, public libraries were prized. Open to all without restriction, requiring no fees, and lending their collections freely, they were deemed important sources of knowledge to inform a literate and thoughtful citizenry. Though often funded by taxes, libraries benefited most significantly from their greatest private supporter, steel tycoon Andrew Carnegie. A self-educated Scottish immigrant, Carnegie spent $60 million to fund libraries. Though a ruthless businessman who refused to accede to workers' demands for higher pay, he believed that knowledge, not money, was the currency of value (as perhaps only a very wealthy man can believe). Carnegie lived by his statement that "the man who dies rich dies in disgrace." His first commissioned library was in his home town of Allegheny, Pennsylvania, followed by others in Pittsburgh. The Carnegie library in Washington, D.C., the city's oldest, bears over its entrance the motto "Dedicated to the diffusion of knowledge." Before he died in 1919, Carnegie built 1,689 libraries throughout the United States, which served hard-scrabble farmers and miners as well as middle-class and affluent patrons.

34. Which of the following provides the best summary of the passage?

(A) A self-educated man, Andrew Carnegie lived by a motto that required him to give away most of his money.
(B) As a ruthless tycoon, Carnegie believed that the accumulation of wealth was the most important endeavor in the young democracy.
(C) Public libraries, which are important resources for educating people in a democracy, benefited greatly from Andrew Carnegie's library funding.
(D) Andrew Carnegie subscribed to the idea that free libraries, open to all, are the foundation of a thriving democracy.

35. The primary purpose of the author's reference to the Washington, D.C., library is

(A) to serve as an example of Carnegie's support for libraries.
(B) to provide evidence for Carnegie's desire to beautify the nation's capital.
(C) to explain the importance of libraries to a young nation.
(D) to underscore the need for free access to public buildings.

36. Which of the following presents events in Andrew Carnegie's life in the correct order?

(A) Becomes wealthy; returns to Scotland; builds the Washington, D.C., library
(B) Immigrates from Scotland; becomes wealthy; builds the Allegheny library
(C) Builds the Washington, D.C., library; builds libraries in Pennsylvania; builds the Allegheny library
(D) Immigrates from Scotland; builds the Washington, D.C., library; builds the Allegheny library

37. What can be inferred about the author's point of view from the comment that Carnegie prized knowledge over money "as perhaps only a very wealthy man can believe"?

(A) Knowledge is always more important than money.
(B) Carnegie was hypocritical in amassing wealth.
(C) Carnegie misunderstood the importance of money.
(D) The very wealthy can afford to downplay the importance of money.

38. According to the passage, what is the most important characteristic of libraries?

(A) There were over a thousand free libraries by 1919.
(B) They provide needed information for knowledgeable citizens.
(C) They are always funded by taxes.
(D) They lend materials without restriction.

Questions 39–40 are based on the following passage.

There are three European professional cycling stage races in the Grand Tour: Giro d'Italia, Tour de France, and Vuelta a España. The oldest and most enjoyable is the Tour de France, first held in 1903 and usually taking place in July. Originally launched to promote a sports newspaper, it is now the most famous bicycle race in the world. The Giro d'Italia and Vuelta a España are held to be almost as prestigious by professional cyclists and the sport's fans, and together the three races make up the Grand Tour of professional race cycling. The Giro d'Italia was originally mounted a few years after the first Tour de France to promote the newspaper *Gazzetta dello Sport*, but the Vuelta a España first ran in 1935. Originally run in April, not long before the Giro d'Italia, the Vuelta a España now takes place in the fall.

39. In which sentence does the author make a value judgment?

   (A) The first sentence
   (B) The second sentence
   (C) The fourth sentence
   (D) The author makes no value judgments.

40. Which is the current annual sequence for the races that make up the Grand Tour?

   (A) Tour de France, Giro d'Italia, Vuelta a España
   (B) Giro d'Italia, Tour de France, Vuelta a España
   (C) Vuelta a España, Giro d'Italia, Tour de France
   (D) Vuelta a España, Tour de France, Giro d'Italia

Marcus should have been happy on his wedding day, but he looked dolefully toward the chapel door for his bride-to-be.

41. Which of the following is the meaning of "dolefully" as used in the sentence?

   (A) Eagerly
   (B) Joyously
   (C) Sadly
   (D) Warily

Questions 42–43 are based on the following story.

Jovian Mining

"What's the old man like?" Buck asked, as Cole fiddled with the old radio.

"Like all the other damn fools who come out two billion miles to scratch rock, as if there weren't enough already on the inner planets. He's got a rich platinum property. Sells 90 percent of his output to buy his power, and the other 11 percent for his clothes and food."

"He must be an efficient miner, to maintain 101 percent production like that."

"No, but his bank account is. He's figured out that's the most economic level of production. If he produces less, he won't be able to pay for his heating power, and if he produces more, his operation will burn up his bank account too fast."

"I take it he's not after money—just the fun," suggested Buck.

"Oh, no. He's after money," replied Cole gravely. "You ask him—he's going to make his eternal fortune yet by striking a real bed of jovium, and then he'll retire."

"Oh, one of that kind."

"They all are," Cole laughed. "Eternal hope, and the rest of it."

Source: Excerpted from *The Ultimate Weapon*, by John W. Campbell, 1936. This work is in the public domain.

42. What is the main idea that emerges in Buck and Cole's conversation?

   (A) Miners are practical in the everyday details of their work but have wildly optimistic dreams of making their fortune.
   (B) Only the desperate and foolish become miners, especially on the outer planets.
   (C) The misunderstood miner is a romantic frontiersman, only interested in the adventure.
   (D) Hard and steady work will eventually pay off.

43. It can be inferred from the passage that

   (A) most miners eventually lose all their money.
   (B) Buck and Cole look down on the miners.
   (C) jovium is both rarer and more valuable than platinum.
   (D) Buck and Cole have been working together for years.

A wise man once said that you can lead a child to school but you can't make him learn. It's long been established that a person's grit—that is, their perseverance, their confidence, and their endurance—is the greatest predictor of their future success. Yet parents spend a fortune on expensive prep schools and colleges they can hardly afford for kids who refuse to break a sweat. They would be better off sending their kids to military boot camp first and college second. It would be cheaper, and all those push-ups might actually help a kid lift those oh-so-heavy textbook covers.

44. Based on this passage, what underlying belief does the author have?

(A) Military training helps build "grit."
(B) Being accepted to college is a good indicator that a student is a diligent, self-reliant learner.
(C) Students with "grit" don't need to do as much reading in college courses as their classmates with less character.
(D) Parents who spend a lot of money on their children's education make the children lazy.

Questions 45–46 are based on the following postcard.

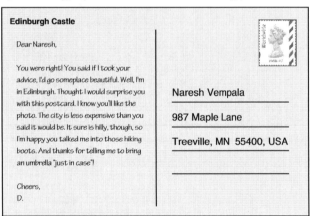

Edinburgh Castle

Dear Naresh,

You were right! You said if I took your advice, I'd go someplace beautiful. Well, I'm in Edinburgh. Thought I would surprise you with this postcard. I know you'll like the photo. The city is less expensive than you said it would be. It sure is hilly, though, so I'm happy you talked me into those hiking boots. And thanks for telling me to bring an umbrella "just in case"!

Cheers,
D.

Naresh Vempala

987 Maple Lane

Treeville, MN 55400, USA

45. Which of the following is a piece of advice that the author did NOT get from Naresh?

(A) Bring an umbrella.
(B) Wear hiking boots.
(C) Visit Edinburgh.
(D) Buy a photo postcard of Edinburgh Castle.

46. Which of the following questions would the postcard writer have logically asked in order to reach a conclusion based on Naresh's advice?

(A) Is Edinburgh a beautiful city?
(B) Is Edinburgh Castle an impressive structure?
(C) Will Naresh enjoy receiving a postcard?
(D) Are there less expensive places to visit than Edinburgh?

The night before a workday, I set my alarm for 8:00 AM after I make sure my watch battery is charged. In the morning, when my alarm rings, I hit the snooze button to get 10 extra minutes of blissful sleep. After the alarm rings for the second time, I make a mental checklist of things I have to do at work and any plans I've made for after work. Then it's time to start my day.

47. What does the author of the passage state is the first step in preparing for the workday?

(A) "I set my alarm for 8:00 AM."
(B) "I hit the snooze button."
(C) "I make a mental checklist of things I have to do at work."
(D) "I make sure my watch battery is charged."

Questions 48–49 are based on the following passage.

The media are really out of control. When the press gets a story, it seems that within minutes it has produced flashy moving graphics and sound effects to entice viewers and garner ratings. Real facts and unbiased coverage of an issue are totally abandoned in exchange for an overly sentimental or one-sided story that too often distorts the truth. Unless viewers learn to recognize real reporting from the junk on nearly every television channel these days, they will be badly misinformed about current events.

48. In this passage, the author refers to graphics and sound effects in order to

(A) give examples of features that make news reports more interesting and relevant.
(B) define through specific examples what he means by "junk."
(C) draw a distinction between biased and neutral reporting.
(D) illustrate ways in which the media depart from unbiased news reporting.

49. The author's primary purpose in writing this passage is to

(A) criticize indiscriminate television viewers.
(B) support the use of graphics and sound effects to add interest to a news report.
(C) distinguish between biased and neutral news reporting.
(D) condemn the media for distorting news reports.

Questions 50–51 are based on the following passage.

The first passage below is a newspaper article about recent legislation. The second is a letter to the editor of that newspaper in response to the legislation.

New Tractor License Requirements

State senators narrowly passed a bill last week that will require minors to have their tractor license (available at the age of 14 1/2 in this state) when working the land with heavy equipment, even on their own family's farms. Prior to this bill's passing, a license was only required when operating a tractor on public rural roads, necessary only when crossing from one field to another. The bill's sponsors argued that while state laws permit children to work in a family business when they would be too young to work under other circumstances, it's necessary to take special steps to protect minors from potentially dangerous work. The bill, which was passed as a Child Labor Law amendment and not part of the Highway Traffic Act, will prevent children too young to hold a tractor license from operating heavy equipment, though not from working on their family farm.

Thanks for "Taking Care" of Us

I was so pleased to read about how the state senators, desperate for something to do with their time, decided to start adding more restrictions on how struggling farmers can run their business. There have been farmers here longer than there have been state senators, and I should know: my family homesteaded in this county almost two hundred years ago, and we've always taken good care of our kids. But please, by all means, tell us how to raise our children and put food on *your* table, all while ignoring the economic realities of this industry. One season after another, we keep getting asked to do more with less, and we'll keep doing it. Until one day we can't. But I'm sure the state senate will find a way to bail us out. They're so good at dealing with nonexistent problems, they've probably gotten all the practice they need to deal with the real ones they've created.

50. What is the main point of disagreement between the farmer who wrote the response to the news story and the state officials who sponsored and approved the bill?

(A) The state senators want to restrict all children under the age of 14 1/2 from working, while the farmer claims that family-owned businesses need this labor.

(B) The farmer disagrees with the state senators' assumptions about safety issues in child farm labor.

(C) The state senators and the farmer disagree about whether children's safety or farming families' economic security should be a higher priority.

(D) The state senators argue that there is high risk of injury to children from farmwork, while the farmer claims the danger lies only in operating heavy equipment.

51. The farmer who wrote the response to the news article apparently believes that

(A) this bill will make operating farms more difficult for families by preventing them from hiring neighborhood children for lower wages.

(B) the state is actively trying to destroy the agriculture industry.

(C) minor injuries are all part of a day's work and this is a lesson children should learn.

(D) the state overestimates the danger to children of operating tractors.

There are five species of frigate birds, a family of seabirds found across tropical and subtropical oceans. Three of the species are widespread, _____ two are endangered with restricted breeding habitats.

52. Which of the following words best completes the blank?

(A) while
(B) therefore
(C) consequently
(D) because

Fortunately, the election campaign has seen a shift from pejorative vilification to constructive debate in the last few weeks.

53. Which of the following words has a positive connotation as used here?

(A) shift
(B) pejorative
(C) vilification
(D) constructive

IF YOU FINISH BEFORE TIME IS CALLED, YOU MAY CHECK YOUR WORK ON THIS SECTION ONLY. DO NOT TURN TO ANY OTHER SECTION IN THE TEST.

STOP

Mathematics

Directions You have 54 minutes to answer 36 questions. Do not work on any other section of the test during this time. You may use a four-function calculator for this section of the test only.

1. What is the decimal equivalent of 4.5%?

   (A) 0.0045
   (B) 0.045
   (C) 0.45
   (D) 4.5

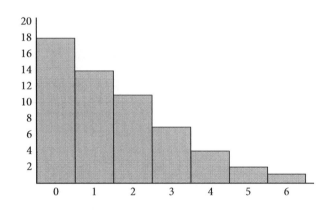

2. Which of the following correctly describes the distribution portrayed by the above graph?

   (A) Skewed right
   (B) Skewed left
   (C) Normal
   (D) Symmetrical

3. $4y + 36 = 128$

   Solve for y in the equation above. Which of the following is correct?

   (A) 23
   (B) 41
   (C) 92
   (D) 164

4. A restaurant worker is cutting oranges. He cuts each orange into six slices and can cut up one orange every 15 seconds. If he maintains this rate, how many slices will he create in 15 minutes?

   (A) 60
   (B) 90
   (C) 225
   (D) 360

5. A study conducted early in the 20th century found that the more telephones that were present in a household, the higher the incidence of cancer. Which of the following must be true about the relationship between telephones and cancer based on the results of the study?

   (A) There was a positive covariance between the number of telephones and the incidence of cancer.
   (B) There was a negative covariance between the number of telephones and the incidence of cancer.
   (C) There was no cause and effect relationship between telephones and cancer.
   (D) Talking on the telephone causes cancer.

6. There are marbles of four different colors in a bag. The ratio of red to white to blue marbles is 3:4:5. There are half as many green marbles as there are blue marbles. What is the least possible number of marbles in the bag?

   (A) 12
   (B) 24
   (C) 29
   (D) 58

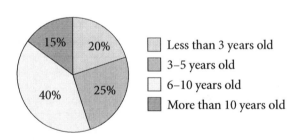

7. A fruit orchard has 300 apple trees. The chart above shows the distribution of ages of the apple trees. How many apple trees are 5 years old or younger?

   (A) 45
   (B) 75
   (C) 135
   (D) 165

8. The children at a nursery school are painting eggs for a holiday party. They paint a total of 30 eggs. They paint 5 of the eggs blue, 5 of the eggs yellow, 5 of the eggs pink, and the remaining eggs green. What fraction of the eggs are painted green?

(A) $\dfrac{1}{15}$

(B) $\dfrac{1}{6}$

(C) $\dfrac{5}{15}$

(D) $\dfrac{1}{2}$

9. What is the value of $27 \times 47 \times 31 \times 61$?

(A) 2,399,679
(B) 2,401,775
(C) 2,403,094
(D) 2,405,353

10. $1\dfrac{7}{8} \times 3\dfrac{1}{5}$

Simplify the expression above.

(A) $\dfrac{21}{40}$

(B) $\dfrac{4}{5}$

(C) $3\dfrac{7}{40}$

(D) 6

11. A physical therapist is using a wide elastic band to help a patient strengthen his knee after surgery. At the patient's current stage of therapy, he should not exert more than 20 kilograms weight of force. The band being used for this therapy exerts a force of 40 grams of weight for every millimeter it is extended. The relationship between force applied and the distance the band is extended is linear. What is the maximum distance the therapist should allow the patient to extend the band?

(A) 5 millimeters
(B) 5 centimeters
(C) 5 decimeters
(D) 80 centimeters

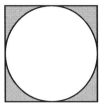

12. A circle is inscribed in a square as shown in the figure above. If the side length of the square is 6 inches, what is the area of the shaded region, in square inches?

(A) $36 - 9\pi$
(B) $36 - 6\pi$
(C) $36 + 6\pi$
(D) $36 - 3\pi$

13. $4, 3.35, \dfrac{11}{3}, \dfrac{13}{4}, \dfrac{7}{2}$

Order the numbers above from least to greatest.

(A) $\dfrac{7}{2}, \dfrac{11}{3}, \dfrac{13}{4}, 3.35, 4$

(B) $\dfrac{13}{4}, 3.35, \dfrac{7}{2}, \dfrac{11}{3}, 4$

(C) $4, 3.35, \dfrac{13}{4}, \dfrac{11}{3}, \dfrac{7}{2}$

(D) $4, \dfrac{11}{3}, \dfrac{7}{2}, 3.35, \dfrac{13}{4}$

14. A nurse in a postsurgical ward records the blood pressure of a certain client no fewer than 2 times per hour and no more than 6 times per hour. Which expression describes the number of times, n, that the nurse will record the client's blood pressure in an 8-hour shift?

(A) $8 \le n \le 48$
(B) $16 \le n \le 48$
(C) $16 \ge n \ge 48$
(D) $16 \le n \le 64$

15. A personal trainer produces her own brand of sports drink to distribute to her clients. She produces the drink by diluting a commercial nutrient mix into a 15 percent concentrated solution. The commercial nutrient mix is sold by the bottle, in bottles containing 10 ounces each. How many bottles of the nutrient mix will the trainer need to buy to produce 240 ounces of her sports drink?

(A) 3
(B) 4
(C) 24
(D) 36

16. $\dfrac{7}{8}+\dfrac{5}{6}+\dfrac{3}{4}$

    Simplify the expression above.

    (A) $\dfrac{5}{8}$

    (B) $\dfrac{5}{6}$

    (C) $2\dfrac{5}{12}$

    (D) $2\dfrac{11}{24}$

17. If the ratio of a to b is 4 to 3 and the ratio of b to c is 1 to 5, what is the ratio of a to c?

    (A) $\dfrac{4}{15}$

    (B) $\dfrac{1}{3}$

    (C) $\dfrac{2}{5}$

    (D) $\dfrac{4}{5}$

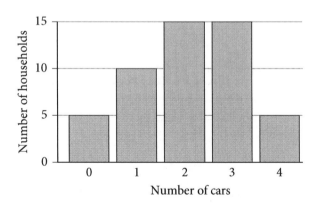

18. The bar graph above shows the number of cars owned per household for 50 households. According to the graph, how many households own at least three cars?

    (A) 4
    (B) 5
    (C) 15
    (D) 20

19. $917 \div 31 \times 4$

    What is the value of the expression above, rounded to the nearest whole number?
    (A) 70
    (B) 94
    (C) 118
    (D) 152

20. A fuel tank initially contains 180 L of fuel. After 360 L are added, the tank is $\dfrac{5}{8}$ full. What is the total capacity of the tank?

    (A) 576 L
    (B) 864 L
    (C) 1000 L
    (D) 1244 L

21. How many milligrams are in 2 kilograms?

    (A) 2,000,000
    (B) 200,000
    (C) 20,000
    (D) 2,000

22. In the following equations, the variable p is independent and q is dependent. In which equation is the relationship between p and q positively covariant?

    (A) $q = p^2 + 4$
    (B) $q = p + 4 - p$
    (C) $q = p + 4$
    (D) $q = 4 - p$

23. Which of the following expressions is equal to

    $6a + \dfrac{4(a-8)}{2} + a + 1$?

    (A) $6a + 33$
    (B) $9a - 15$
    (C) $9a - 31$
    (D) $11a + 17$

24. A bicyclist regularly travels the same route during training for a race. There are three segments on this route: an uphill segment, a level segment, and a downhill segment. On the uphill segment, the bicyclist travels at 15 mph and covers the distance in 20 minutes. On the level segment, she travels at 20 mph and covers the distance in 1 hour. On the downhill segment, she travels at 30 mph. If the entire trip takes her 2 hours to complete, what is the distance of all three segments combined?

    (A) 32.5 miles
    (B) 45 miles
    (C) 65 miles
    (D) 95 miles

25. Janice received a large bonus, so she treated her friends to lunch at a local restaurant. The total price for the food and beverages was $110.50 before sales tax was added. Later, when Janice was reviewing her monthly charge card statement, she noticed that the total amount she had paid, including the tip and 6% sales tax, was an even $140. Rounded to the nearest tenth, what percentage of the price plus tax was the tip that Janice left for the server?

   (A) 15.0%
   (B) 19.5%
   (C) 20.7%
   (D) 26.7%

26. $2 \times (8 \times 10 - 5) + 5$

   What is the value of the expression above?

   (A) 85
   (B) 155
   (C) 160
   (D) 165

27. A gardener plants a 60-square-foot vegetable garden with carrot seeds and lettuce seeds. In each square foot of the garden, he plants either 6 carrot seeds or 2 lettuce seeds. If he plants two-thirds of the area of the garden with carrot seeds, and the remaining area with lettuce seeds, what is the ratio of lettuce seeds to carrot seeds?

   (A) 6:1
   (B) 1:2
   (C) 1:3
   (D) 1:6

28. April purchased a bottle of spring water on her way to work. After her morning break, she noticed that she had consumed $\frac{2}{7}$ of her water. After her afternoon break, $\frac{1}{3}$ of the water remained. Approximately what was the percentage change in the amount of water left in April's bottle between the two times that she noted the level of the bottle's contents?

   (A) 53%
   (B) 27%
   (C) −53%
   (D) −71%

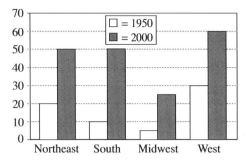

29. The bar graph above shows the number of clinics in different regions in the years 1950 and 2000. What was the average of the number of clinics in the South and West in 1950?

   (A) 10
   (B) 20
   (C) 40
   (D) 55

30. At a pharmacy, the ratio of containers of a brand-name prescription medicine to the generic version of that medicine is 7:2. If the pharmacy adds 6 more containers of the generic version to its inventory, the ratio becomes 11:4. What was the original total number of containers of the two medicines in stock?

   (A) 11
   (B) 22
   (C) 77
   (D) 99

31. $3 + 5 \times (8 + 4) \div 3 - 7$

   What is the value of the expression above?

   (A) 14
   (B) 16
   (C) 25
   (D) 30

32. $3m - 15 = \frac{m}{2} + 110$

   Solve for m in the equation above. Which of the following is correct?

   (A) 25
   (B) 38
   (C) 50
   (D) 125

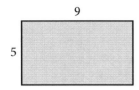

33. What is the area, in square units, of a square that has the same perimeter as the rectangle above?

    (A) 25
    (B) 36
    (C) 49
    (D) 64

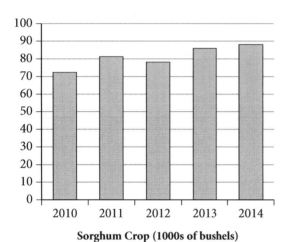

Sorghum Crop (1000s of bushels)

34. The graph above shows a farm's production of sorghum by year. The acreage devoted to sorghum was cut significantly in 2015, and, as a result, that year's sorghum crop was half that of 2012's production. How much sorghum was produced in 2015?

    (A) 36,000 bushels
    (B) 39,000 bushels
    (C) 40,000 bushels
    (D) 42,000 bushels

35. Approximately how many ounces are in four kilograms? (Note: 1 kilogram ≈ 2.2 pounds and 1 pound = 16 ounces.)

    (A) 140.8
    (B) 35.2
    (C) 29.1
    (D) 7.3

36. Jan is a pet sitter who wants to build a kennel and a dog run in her yard. The kennel will be a square enclosure 9 feet on a side, and the dog run will be a rectangular enclosure 6 feet wide by 20 feet long. If she wants to completely fence each enclosure, what is the total length of fencing Jan will need?

    (A) 38 feet
    (B) 62 feet
    (C) 64 feet
    (D) 88 feet

IF YOU FINISH BEFORE TIME IS CALLED, YOU MAY CHECK YOUR WORK ON THIS SECTION ONLY. DO NOT TURN TO ANY OTHER SECTION IN THE TEST. YOU MAY NOW TAKE A 10-MINUTE BREAK. STOP

Science

Directions You have 63 minutes to answer 53 questions. Do not work on any other section of the test during this time.

1. Which of the following are parts of a neuron?

   (A) Brain, spinal column, and nerve cells
   (B) Autonomic and somatic
   (C) Dendrites, axon, and soma
   (D) Sympathetic and parasympathetic

2. Which of the following organelles is NOT involved in protein translation or processing?

   (A) Ribosome
   (B) Rough ER
   (C) Mitochondrion
   (D) Golgi apparatus

3. Which of the following is primarily absorbed in the ileum?

   (A) Vitamin K
   (B) Carbohydrates
   (C) Water
   (D) Vitamin B_{12}

4. Which of the following correctly includes all the layers of the skin, from the deepest layer outward?

   (A) hypodermis, dermis, epidermis
   (B) subcutaneous, sebaceous, dermis
   (C) sebaceous, epidermis, dermis
   (D) dermis, hypodermis, epidermis

5. Which of the following is NOT a possible pairing of period numbers and orbital names?

   (A) 2 and d
   (B) 3 and d
   (C) 2 and s
   (D) 2 and p

6. Which of the following is NOT a possible consequence of hypertension?

   (A) Vascular scarring from increased plaque buildup
   (B) Hemoglobin not properly binding to oxygen
   (C) Stroke or aneurysm resulting from blood clots
   (D) Heart or kidney failure from poor vascularization

7. Which of the following is NOT a function of the kidney?

   (A) Filtering blood
   (B) Maintaining blood pressure
   (C) Activating vitamin D
   (D) Storing urea

8. How many milligrams are in 10 grams?

   (A) 100 mg
   (B) 1000 mg
   (C) 10,000 mg
   (D) 100,000 mg

9. In which of the following would blood pressure be the highest?

   (A) Aorta
   (B) Capillaries
   (C) Pulmonary arteries
   (D) Vena cava

Questions 10—12 are based on the following diagram.

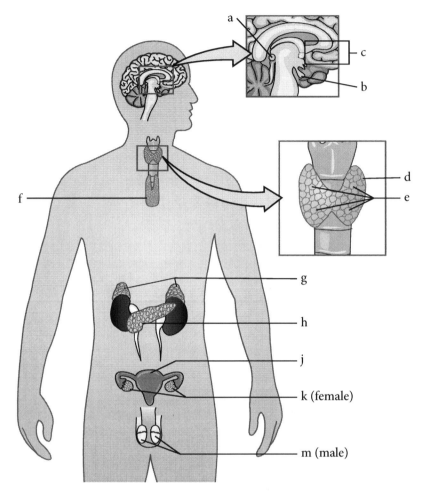

Each letter in the diagram corresponds to a specific anatomical body part. Use the letters above to answer the following questions.

10. Which of the following secretes the hormone that regulates sleep cycle?

    (A) a
    (B) d
    (C) f
    (D) g

11. Which of the following is stimulated to release hormones by an electrical signal?

    (A) b
    (B) c
    (C) e
    (D) k

12. In which of the following would progesterone be produced in response to a surge of luteinizing hormone (LH)?

    (A) b
    (B) j
    (C) k
    (D) m

13. Which of the following is NOT a function of surfactant in the lungs?

    (A) Prevent alveolar collapse
    (B) Increase gas exchange
    (C) Decrease gas exchange
    (D) Decrease surface tension

14. Which of the following correctly describes the sequence of chemical digestion in the stomach?

    (A) Glucagon stimulates the release of gastric juice.
    (B) Gherlin stimulates the release of HCl and pepsin.
    (C) Gastrin stimulates the release of HCl and pepsinogen.
    (D) Goblet cells stimulate the release of pepsin and pepsinogen.

15. Which of the following are responsible for transmitting a motor impulse across the neuromuscular junction?

    (A) Neurotransmitters
    (B) Nodes of Ranvier
    (C) Calcium ions
    (D) Action potentials

16. When the body temperature becomes abnormally high, which of the following homeostatic processes occurs?

    (A) Sweat gland activity and blood flow to the subcutaneous layer of the skin increase, and hair follicles relax.
    (B) Sweat gland activity and blood flow to the subcutaneous layer of the skin increase, and hair follicles contract.
    (C) Sweat gland activity increases, blood flow to the subcutaneous layer of the skin decreases, and hair follicles relax.
    (D) Sweat gland activity decreases, blood flow to the subcutaneous layer of the skin increases, and hair follicles relax.

17. Which of the following is an enzyme that regulates arterial blood pressure?

    (A) Epinephrine
    (B) Renin
    (C) Glucagon
    (D) Nephron

18. Which of the following physical properties changes when volume changes but mass is held constant?

    (A) Electronegativity
    (B) Density
    (C) Atomic radius
    (D) First ionization energy

19. Which of the following could result when the body is exposed to a live pathogen?

    (A) Active immunity
    (B) Passive immunity
    (C) Antigen resistance
    (D) Autoimmune disease

20. A person complains of sciatica, pain that shoots from the lower back through the hips and legs. What is the most likely cause?

    (A) Herniated lumbar disc
    (B) Fractured coccyx
    (C) Bruised calf muscle
    (D) Myocardial infarction

21. A recent editorial critical of a political candidate alleged, among other things, that she is more popular with less educated voters than with those with more education. The candidate believes that she is equally popular among voters across all levels of education. Her campaign manager wants to conduct a poll to ascertain which belief is correct. What would be an appropriate null hypothesis to test with the poll?

    (A) The candidate is more popular among voters with less education than voters with more education.
    (B) Other candidates are more popular among voters with more education.
    (C) There is no correlation between the candidate's popularity and voters' income levels.
    (D) There is no correlation between the candidate's popularity and voters' education.

22. Which of the following is NOT found in smooth muscle?

    (A) Actin
    (B) Myosin
    (C) Sarcomere
    (D) Gap junction

Questions 23–25 are based on the following information.

For most substances, the solid phase is the densest, with molecules tightly packed in an orderly pattern. Water is the only substance that is denser as a liquid than as a solid and, as a result, has special properties. The phase diagram of water is shown below.

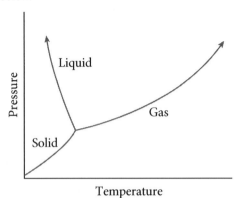

A scientist set out to determine how the presence of contaminants in water changed its freezing point. The scientist added increasing concentrations of sodium chloride to water and measured the freezing point of each solution. The results are summarized in the following table.

Solution Composition	Freezing Point (°C)
Pure Water	0
1M	−2
2M	−4
3M	−6

Experimental Results

23. What would eventually happen to solid ice when the pressure is significantly increased at constant temperature?

   (A) It would become a denser form of ice.
   (B) It would melt to form the less dense liquid state.
   (C) It would melt to form the denser liquid state.
   (D) There would be no change.

24. Which of the following is a valid conclusion that can be made from the freezing point data?

   (A) Salt increases the freezing point of water, enabling it to melt at higher temperatures.
   (B) Salt decreases the freezing point of water, enabling it to melt at higher temperatures.
   (C) Salt decreases the freezing point of water, enabling it to melt at lower temperatures.
   (D) Salt increases the freezing point of water, enabling it to melt at lower temperatures.

25. Which of the following is NOT an endothermic process?

   (A) Melting
   (B) Sublimation
   (C) Vaporization
   (D) Deposition

26. In its final stage, the HIV virus disrupts the immune system by which of the following methods?

   (A) Destroying lymphocytic cells that contain an antigen signature
   (B) Favoring the production of memory cells over immunoglobulins
   (C) Overproducing IgE and triggering a histamine reaction
   (D) Preventing the activation of cytotoxic T-cells

27. Which of the following correctly describes the role of the integumentary system?

   (A) Maintains adequate blood volume
   (B) Protects the body against dehydration
   (C) Secretes hormones into the bloodstream
   (D) Expels excess fluid from the body

28. The price of a call option at any point in time depends upon, among other factors, the number of days remaining until the option expires and the price of the underlying stock upon which the option is based. Some representative values are shown in the following table.

Days Remaining	Stock Price	Call Price
30	$20.00	$1.00
60	$20.00	$1.75
90	$20.00	$2.00
30	$40.00	$2.00
60	$40.00	$3.50
90	$40.00	$4.00
30	$60.00	$3.00
60	$60.00	$5.25
90	$60.00	$6.00

Which of the following is true based on the relationships that can be determined from the data in the table?

(A) Call prices are unrelated to either stock prices or days remaining.
(B) Call prices are positively, linearly related to both stock prices and days remaining.
(C) Call prices are positively, linearly related to stock prices and positively, but not linearly, related to days remaining.
(D) Call prices are positively, but not linearly, related to stock prices and positively, linearly related to days remaining.

29. Which of the following correctly identifies the location of the sternum on the body?

(A) Superior and ventral
(B) Superior and dorsal
(C) Inferior and ventral
(D) Inferior and dorsal

30. Under normal circumstances, which of the following is normally found in urine?

(A) Glucose
(B) Urea
(C) Blood cells
(D) Amino acids

31. Which of the following statements is true of ventricular systole?

(A) The ventricles relax and are passively filled with blood.
(B) The ventricles are forcibly filled with blood from the atria.
(C) The semilunar valves open under increased pressure.
(D) The atrioventricular (AV) valves open under increased pressure

32. A researcher found that 17 percent of people suffering from chronic pain described themselves as very unhappy with their lives and 30 percent said they were somewhat unhappy. When he studied a group of people with the same demographic characteristics who were not experiencing chronic pain, only 6 percent said they were very unhappy with their lives and 17 percent were somewhat unhappy. Based on the results of his study, the researcher concluded that unhappiness is a major cause of chronic pain. Which of the following errors did the researcher make in reaching his conclusion?

(A) He equated correlation with causation.
(B) The study was biased.
(C) He only performed one study.
(D) He did not have a null hypothesis.

33. Which of the following nervous systems work in tandem to maintain homeostasis of the body?

(A) Central and peripheral
(B) Autonomic and sympathetic
(C) Somatic and autonomic
(D) Sympathetic and parasympathetic

34. Which of the following involves chemical digestion?

(A) Salivating
(B) Swallowing
(C) Chewing
(D) Belching

35. Which of the following is NOT composed of macromolecules?

(A) Carbohydrate
(B) Gastric acid
(C) Nucleic acid
(D) Lipid

36. Homeostatic control of blood glucose by insulin and glucagon is achieved by which of the following?

    (A) A decrease in blood glucose stimulates glucagon; an increase in blood glucose stimulates insulin.
    (B) An increase in insulin lowers blood glucose; an increase in blood glucose stimulates glucagon.
    (C) A increase in blood glucose stimulates glucagon; a decrease in blood glucose stimulates insulin.
    (D) An increase in glucagon lowers blood glucose; a decrease in insulin lowers blood glucose.

37. Balance the chemical equation

    ____ $Hg(OH)_2$ + ____ H_3PO_4 → $Hg_3(PO_4)_2$ + ____ H_2O

    by identifying the coefficients that correctly fill in the blanks.

    (A) 2, 3, 6
    (B) 3, 2, 6
    (C) 3, 2, 8
    (D) 6, 4, 12

38. Which of the following is a short bone?

    (A) Phalange
    (B) Tarsal
    (C) Scapula
    (D) Radius

39. Which hormone is responsible for triggering ovulation?

    (A) Luteinizing hormone
    (B) Estrogen
    (C) Corpus luteum
    (D) Progesterone

40. Which of the following would decrease the rate of diffusion of oxygen from the lungs into the bloodstream?

    (A) Decreasing the concentration of oxygen in the blood
    (B) Increasing the surface area of the alveoli
    (C) Increasing the concentration of carbon dioxide in the blood
    (D) Increasing the concentration of oxygen in the blood

41. The prescribed dose of a certain medication is 1 deciliter. The amount administered must be accurate to within ±1 percent. The amount being administered should be measured in what unit to the nearest whole number to ensure that the needed accuracy is attained?

    (A) Decaliters
    (B) Deciliters
    (C) Milliliters
    (D) Microliters

42. Which of the following produces bile?

    (A) Gall bladder
    (B) Bile duct
    (C) Duodenum
    (D) Liver

43. Which of the following correctly pairs the reproductive structure with its function?

    (A) Fallopian tubes, site of fertilization
    (B) Prostate gland, produces sperm
    (C) Uterus, site of fertilization
    (D) Testes, produces nourishing fluid for sperm

44. White fur is a recessive trait in a certain species of mammal. A black-furred parent and a white-furred parent produce an offspring that has white fur. Which of the following deductions is supported by the information given?

    (A) The parents' next offspring will be black.
    (B) The white-furred parent has a recessive black fur allele.
    (C) The black-furred parent has a recessive white fur allele.
    (D) The offspring has one black fur allele and one white fur allele.

45. Which of the following blood vessels contain valves to prevent blood from flowing backward?

    (A) Arteries
    (B) Capillaries
    (C) Ventricles
    (D) Veins

46. Ohm's law states that $V = IR$, where V is voltage, I is current flow, and R is total resistance. A science class performs an experiment to determine how placing two different resistors, with resistance r_1 and r_2, in parallel affects the total resistance of a circuit. The experiment uses a constant voltage; as the different resistors are placed in parallel in the circuit, the current flow is measured. From these values of V and I, R can be calculated using the proven logic of Ohm's law. Which of the following equations is a hypothesis that can be evaluated with this experiment?

(A) $V = IR$

(B) $R = \dfrac{r_1 r_2}{r_1 + r_2}$

(C) $R = \dfrac{V}{I}$

(D) $r_1 = \dfrac{R \times r_2}{r_2 + R}$

47. Which of the following statements correctly describes the contraction of muscles and change in pressure inside the lungs during inhalation?

(A) The diaphragm and intercostal muscles contract, decreasing pressure in the lungs.
(B) The diaphragm and intercostal muscles contract, increasing pressure in the lungs.
(C) The diaphragm and intercostal muscles relax, increasing pressure in the lungs
(D) The diaphragm and intercostal muscles relax, decreasing pressure in the lungs.

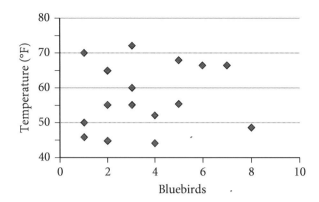

48. A birder records the number of bluebirds he spotted on any given day and the high temperature recorded that day, as shown on the scatterplot above. Which of the following best describes the relationship between the temperature and the number of bluebirds observed based on the data shown?

(A) The number of bluebirds observed correlates positively with temperature.
(B) The number of bluebirds observed correlates negatively with temperature.
(C) There is no apparent correlation between temperature and the number of bluebirds observed.
(D) Temperature is inversely correlated with the number of bluebirds observed.

49. Which of the following cells would NOT be involved in the immune response to a pathogen encountered for the first time?

(A) Macrophages
(B) NK lympocytes
(C) Plasma cells
(D) Dendritic cells

50. Which of the following organs does NOT release a hormone involved in the absorption and/or distribution of nutrients from the digestive tract?

    (A) Stomach
    (B) Pancreas
    (C) Liver
    (D) Small intestine

51. Which of the following is a part of the adaptive immune system?

    (A) Phagocytes
    (B) Inflammation
    (C) Earwax
    (D) T-cells

52. Which if the following would lead to a decrease in respiration rate following the onset of hyperventilation?

    (A) Decrease in blood pH
    (B) Increase in blood pH
    (C) Increase in blood carbon dioxide levels
    (D) Increase in blood oxygen levels

53. Which of the following bone cells is responsible for breaking down bone?

    (A) Osteoclasts
    (B) Osteocytes
    (C) Osteoblasts
    (D) Osteons

IF YOU FINISH BEFORE TIME IS CALLED, YOU MAY CHECK YOUR WORK ON THIS SECTION ONLY. DO NOT TURN TO ANY OTHER SECTION IN THE TEST. STOP

English and Language Usage

Directions You have 28 minutes to answer 28 questions. Do not work on any other section of the test during this time.

1. The art teacher reminded her student to purchase his art supplies _____ a paint brush, palette, easel, and canvas.

   Which of the following punctuation marks correctly completes the sentence?

   (A) .
   (B) :
   (C) ;
   (D) ,

2. David decided to contact the appliance repair company regarding his broken washing machine; although he wanted the machine fixed immediately, he thought it best to request a ballpark figure for the repair fee first.

   Which of the following phrases in the sentence above is informal?

   (A) decided to contact
   (B) fixed immediately
   (C) thought it best
   (D) ballpark figure

3. The famous producers _____ planning to release an exciting new film this upcoming fall.

   Which of the following correctly completes the sentence above?

   (A) are
   (B) is
   (C) will
   (D) be

4. Stella was delighted to see that the children enjoyed there gifts.

   Which of the following corrects an error in the sentence above?

   (A) Change "see" to "sea."
   (B) Change "children" to "childrens."
   (C) Change "enjoyed" to "enjoied."
   (D) Change "there" to "their."

5. At the end of the short-term drug trials, the subjects who had received the medication showed no discernible differences in health outcomes when compared to the subjects who had received the placebo.

   In which of the following would the above sentence most likely appear?

   (A) Letter to the editor
   (B) Short story
   (C) Scientific report
   (D) Advertisement

6. _____ she had left the water running, the sink overflowed onto the floor and into the hallway.

   Which word correctly completes the sentence?

   (A) However
   (B) Because
   (C) Even though
   (D) Unless

7. The researcher <u>disclaimed</u> any knowledge of improper use of funds by his team.

   Which of the following is the meaning of the underlined word in the sentence above?

   (A) Admitted
   (B) Proclaimed
   (C) Blamed
   (D) Denied

8. Which of the following sentences would most likely appear in a novel?

   (A) Walter stepped out of the office building and walked toward his car, careful not to slip on the thin layer of ice that covered the parking lot.
   (B) The suspect was captured close to his home yesterday evening after a neighbor contacted police.
   (C) Our profit margin will continue to increase, provided we implement the customer service initiatives suggested by our relationship management team.
   (D) The leafcutter ant is an unusual species in that it grows its own food to feed its young.

9. Marcus attempted to <u>disentangle</u> the fawn caught in the snare.

Which of the following is the meaning of the underlined word in the sentence above?

(A) Free
(B) Hunt
(C) Observe
(D) Trap

10. The girls' volleyball team will win _____ championship game because each player will play _____ best.

Which of the following pairs of words correctly completes the sentence above?

(A) its ; her
(B) it's ; her
(C) its ; their
(D) it's ; its

11. Which of the following examples is a complex sentence?

(A) A member of the city council has proposed a new ordinance.
(B) Under the new law, parking on city streets would be free on weeknights, and the mayor would have the authority to suspend parking fees on major holidays.
(C) Although free parking might draw more patrons to the downtown stores, the city cannot afford to lose any parking revenue.
(D) The council should vote against the proposed ordinance at this time.

12. Which of the following sentences is an example of incorrect subject-verb agreement?

(A) Jolie and Daniel went to the movies after dinner.
(B) The boy with the extra sandwiches is going to share with the girl who forgot her lunch.
(C) Everyone who lost points on the test have to stay after class.
(D) The cheerleaders holding the banner are leading the crowd in a cheer.

13. **Types of Research Methodologies**

1. Quantitative Methods
   a. Description
   b. Application

2. Qualitative Methods
   a. Description
   b. Application

If the outline above is used to write a paper, which of the following statements is most likely to appear in that paper?

(A) Researchers must choose between two types of research methodology.
(B) Application is a type of description.
(C) Types of research include quantitative and qualitative methodologies.
(D) Quantitative methods are preferable to qualitative methods.

14. Which of the following words is spelled incorrectly?

(A) Reliable
(B) Enjoyable
(C) Complyant
(D) Denial

15. Jarvis dropped the laptop. The laptop was expensive. Then the whole group turned around. Everyone in the cafeteria stared at him.

Which of the following best states the information above in a single sentence?

(A) The expensive laptop was dropped by Jarvis and the whole group of people sitting in the cafeteria turned around and stared.
(B) After Jarvis dropped the expensive laptop, everyone in the cafeteria turned around and stared at him.
(C) The laptop, which was expensive, was dropped by Jarvis, and the whole group, who sat in the cafeteria, turned around, staring.
(D) When Jarvis dropped the laptop, then the whole group in the cafeteria turned around and stared at him because it was expensive.

16. Instead of attending the cookout, Ria took a nap because the hot summer weather made her feel lethargic.

As used in the sentence above, "lethargic" most likely means

(A) unfriendly.
(B) bored.
(C) thirsty.
(D) weary.

17. Jessica's abrupt departure left her colleagues in a precarious situation, with no one knowing how to answer the clients' many questions.

As used in the sentence above, "precarious" most likely means

(A) irresponsible.
(B) offensive.
(C) uncertain.
(D) unforeseen.

18. In my opinion, the children at this school have too much freedom, and not nearly enough discipline; for example, they can interrupt the teacher, leave the classroom during lessons, and fail to turn in assignments without facing any repercussions.

Which of the following punctuation marks is used incorrectly in the sentence?

(A) The comma after "opinion"
(B) The comma after "freedom"
(C) The semicolon after "discipline"
(D) The comma after "teacher"

19. Dana did not get dehydrated on her long run because she _____ plenty of water before she began.

Which verb or verb phrase correctly completes the sentence?

(A) drank
(B) had drank
(C) drunk
(D) had drunk

20. The phlebotomist was unable to find suitable _____ in the dehydrated patient's arm.

Which of the following correctly completes the sentence above?

(A) vanes
(B) vains
(C) veins
(D) vein's

21. A clinical trial recently examined the effectiveness of a new beta blocker. The trial tracked patients using the new drug for a period of 18 months and found no serious side effects. All side effects noted were similar in frequency to side effects reported by the control group taking a placebo. Now the trial should be expanded to include more patients and compare this drug's efficacy to that of existing beta blockers available by prescription. Additionally, the trial should explore the use of this beta blocker in comparison with other drugs commonly prescribed for hypertension.

Which of the following sentences would be an appropriate concluding sentence for the paragraph above?

(A) More than 500 patients participated in the clinical study.
(B) The new beta blocker outperformed the placebo on all measures.
(C) Finally, if the expanded trial succeeds, the FDA should consider approving the new drug.
(D) Existing beta blockers do not show similar results in patients over age 35.

22. This summer, my friends are visiting _____ relatives in Europe, and _____ staying for three weeks.

Which of the following pairs of words correctly completes the sentence above?

(A) their ; they're
(B) their ; there
(C) there ; they're
(D) they're ; their

23. Which of the following is the best definition of "prescience"?

(A) Classes taken before a science class
(B) Knowledge of an event before it happens
(C) A written order for medicine
(D) The study of the earth

24. Because Rafael usually enjoys trying new foods, his refusal to visit the restaurant to sample its innovative dishes had his mother scratching her head.

    Which of the following phrases from the sentence is informal?

    (A) trying new foods
    (B) visit the restaurant
    (C) innovative dishes
    (D) scratching her head

25. Gregory trusted Kiera and accepted her offer without reservation.

    As used in the sentence above, "reservation" most likely means

    (A) assignment.
    (B) reliability.
    (C) derivation.
    (D) uncertainty.

26. Which of the following sentences correctly punctuates the dialogue?

    (A) When she found her brother outside, Julie exclaimed, "Michael, there you are! A short while ago, mother said, 'Children, come inside.'"
    (B) When she found her brother outside, Julie exclaimed "Michael, there you are! A short while ago, mother said 'Children, come inside.'"
    (C) When she found her brother outside, Julie exclaimed, "Michael there you are! A short while ago, mother said Children, come inside."
    (D) When she found her brother outside, Julie exclaimed "Michael, there you are! A short while ago, mother said, 'Children, come inside.'"

27. Lack of sleep is more than just an annoyance. A recent study of high school juniors showed that, on average, students who consistently earn low grades go to bed 40 minutes later and get up 25 minutes earlier than students with high grades. _____, another study shows that when a person sleeps less than 6 hours per night, he or she has difficulty remembering information.

    Which of the following words best completes the sentence above?

    (A) Similarly
    (B) However
    (C) Therefore
    (D) In conclusion

28. The rusty old boat with the torn sails is in danger of sinking during the storm.

    Which of the following is the complete subject of the sentence?

    (A) boat
    (B) The rusty old boat
    (C) The rusty old boat with the torn sails
    (D) The rusty old boat with the torn sails is in danger

IF YOU FINISH BEFORE TIME IS CALLED, YOU MAY CHECK YOUR WORK ON THIS SECTION ONLY. DO NOT TURN TO ANY OTHER SECTION IN THE TEST. **STOP**

30 | K

Diagnostic Test Answers and Explanations

Reading

Questions 1–2: Passage Map

Topic: Detective stories
Scope: Relation to public interest in science
Purpose: To explain how rationalism influenced stories
¶ 1: Detective stories written when science very popular
¶ 2: Perception and nature of science different than today
Author: Fictional detectives showed spirit of science

1. **(B) they wrote about heroes whose rational approach mirrored that of real-life scientists.** This question asks for a detail stated in the passage. The first paragraph states that both writers admired scientists and gave their fictional detective characters scientific attitudes and abilities.

2. **(D) out of place.** This is an uncommon word. One clue is the prefix *mal*, which means "bad"; the only answer choice with a negative connotation is **(D)**. If you are not familiar with the prefix, the word's meaning can still be determined from context. Doyle was described as a lover of science, and from context, "rationalist" has a similar meaning. How does ghost hunting fit with scientific thought? Supernatural beliefs tend to involve a different kind of thinking and aren't usually studied scientifically. Also, the next sentence says "these apparent quirks aside," suggesting that this interest seems odd for a man who loves science. So "malapropos" probably means "strange" or "inappropriate." Choice **(D)** is the correct match. Choice (C) might be tempting, because context suggests a possible relationship between "quirky" and "malapropos." However, the tone of the preceding sentence is not positive or admiring, so it doesn't make sense to say that "malapropos" describes a behavior that is endearing.

3. **(B) Courts should stop awarding such excessive settlements.** Sorensen does not make a suggestion in the passage, so to answer this question, you must make an inference. The passage states that Sorensen believes high settlements are a travesty and burden the courts. The rest of the passage explains that these awards set a precedent and provide an incentive for more of these lawsuits. You can infer that Sorensen feels the that the high awards are what lead to a greater workload for the courts. Therefore, predict that he would suggest not awarding such high settlements. Choice **(B)** is a match for that prediction. Choice (A) might seem like a valid inference, since having fewer lawsuits would logically place less of a burden on the courts, but Sorensen's

focus is on the amount of settlements, not on the number of cases brought. Make sure to base your answers to inference questions on the information in the stimulus.

4. **(C) wipe off and replace the drain plug.** According to the passage, "[w]hen the oil is drained fully," you should next wipe off the drain plug and the plug opening and replace the plug. Choice **(C)** is a match for this step in the sequence.

Questions 5–10: Passage Map

Topic: Happiness
Scope: Where it comes from
Purpose: To explain and endorse Haidt's happiness hypothesis
¶ 1: Two theories of happiness: within/without
¶ 2: Haidt: happiness comes from between
Author: Agrees with Haidt

5. **(D) happiness requires a combination of the right internal attitude as well as external life circumstances.** To answer this question about the passage's main idea, use your summary of topic, scope, and purpose. The author endorses Haidt's idea that happiness comes from "between," requiring both internal and external factors. This matches choice **(D)**. The author describes Buddhism and utilitarianism, but the purpose is not to critique them, even though Haidt's hypothesis is presented as correct. Nor is the wisdom of ancient proverbs the main idea, although the passage acknowledges they contain some wisdom that science has confirmed. The statement in answer choice (C) can be inferred from the happiness hypothesis, but this is one aspect of that idea and not the overall focus of the passage.

6. **(A) Utilitarianism** This detail question can be researched in the first paragraph, which discusses several belief systems. Utilitarianism's stance on happiness is briefly defined as the view that "life circumstances happen to satisfy our desires." This is an example of a view that happiness comes from "without," that is, from outside factors rather than from one's own attitude and perception. The question stem's reference to "the state of the world" is another way of saying "without," so utilitarianism, choice **(A)**, is the correct belief system.

7. (D) To provide an example of a belief system in which happiness is held to be influenced by external factors The question asks why the author described utilitarianism in a particular location, so focus on the structure of the passage. The first sentence poses a rhetorical question about where happiness comes from, within or without. This is followed up with examples of belief systems that hold these contrasting views. Utilitarianism is given as the single example of happiness coming from without (based on life circumstances), and it is not mentioned again. Choice **(D)** is therefore the correct answer. Note that this answer choice uses the term "influenced by external factors" instead of "from without." Look for the correct idea in the answer choice; it may be expressed in different words than in the passage.

8. (A) To argue that both internal attitude and life circumstances play a role in a person's happiness To answer this question, you need to determine the author's point of view and purpose in writing. The author goes beyond just explaining the topic, personally showing support for Haidt's happiness hypothesis by saying Haidt "shows" and "establishes" his idea. The author not only describes Haidt's belief in the "between" theory of happiness but argues that Haidt's hypothesis is supported by evidence. Thus, the author's purpose is to argue that Haidt's idea about happiness is correct. While choice (C) also says the author is making an argument, it does not correctly describe the author's point.

9. (B) It would challenge the claim that happiness comes from "without." This question requires you to analyze the effect that new evidence would have on the argument made in the passage. A glance at the answer choices shows that you need to consider how the three points of view described in the passage—happiness comes from within, without, or between—are either supported or undermined by the information given in the question stem. The study says there is a correlation between few material goods and happiness, suggesting that happiness comes more from within than from without. Thus, predict that this evidence would support the within viewpoint and challenge the without and between views. Choice **(B)** is a match for the prediction that the evidence would challenge the without perspective.

10. (B) Because there is more than one way to be happy, even someone in difficult circumstances can find joy with the right outlook. The question asks you to infer which of the answer choices is contrary to the author's point of view. The most specific prediction you can make is that the author agrees with Haidt's "between" hypothesis, so any answer choice that contradicts this hypothesis, including any statement that is based primarily on the "within" or "without" hypotheses, will be correct. Choice **(B)** is based on the "within" hypothesis, saying that external circumstances do

not determine happiness, so the passage author would disagree with this statement. Choices (A) and (C) both state the importance of external and internal factors, and neither choice states that one factor is irrelevant, so they do not contradict the "between" hypothesis. Likewise, choice (D) does not contradict the "between" hypothesis, since it only states that internal factors are related to happiness, not that internal factors are exclusively important.

11. (A) The question presents a hexagon composed of numbered triangles and asks you to follow a series of three instructions. Follow the instructions step-by-step.

1. Switch the positions of numbers 1 and 6.

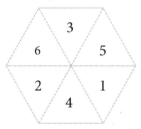

2. Switch the positions of numbers 2 and 5.

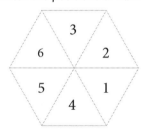

3. Switch the positions of numbers 4 and 5.

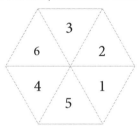

12. (B) Appreciative The author notes that some people have negative feelings toward snakes but uses the key phrase "on the contrary" to introduce some positive attributes snakes possess. Thus, predict a positive word and choose "Appreciative." The author is not disgusted, (A); that would be more appropriate to describe those he disagrees with. Considering the author's appreciation for snakes, it would be incorrect to say he was (C), uninterested, in them. There is no reason to believe that the author is fearful, (D).

13. **(A) January.** The letter writer notes that she lives in the Rocky Mountains and there is currently snow on the ground. Because this is a response to a birthday card, you can conclude that the writer's birthday has occurred recently, and because she lives in the Rocky Mountains, she is in the Northern Hemisphere. Therefore, her birthday occurs during the winter. Of the choices, only January is a winter month.

14. **(B) Contact the Student Association and name some movies by Akira Kurosawa the Association should show.** The question requires you to read the three stimuli and draw a conclusion based on the information you are provided. Jack will not state a preference for Hollywood Horror because *Throne of Blood* is not a horror movie but rather an adaptation of *Macbeth*, a famous quasi-historical tragedy about a Scottish king. He is unlikely to choose English Spy Movies because there is no evidence he is interested in the course on Fleming and le Carré. However, because you know that he is writing a paper on Akira Kurosawa for the Shakespeare Adaptation course, you can infer that he will ask the Student Association to show some movies by Kurosawa so he can bring his experience of watching them to his class.

Questions 15–16: Passage Map

Topic: Toby's transition from childhood
Scope: Baseball as a marker of transition; Toby's last game
Purpose: To tell a story about an important life milestone
¶ 1: Importance of baseball to Toby and his father; Toby soon moving on to adulthood
¶ 2: Anticipation of a good game with dad watching

15. **(A) To tell a story about a significant life milestone** This is a fictional narrative. The author might share his personal beliefs through his characters, but the main goal here is to introduce those characters and tell a story about them.

16. **(D) eager.** Although uneasiness and sadness would be possible answers given the circumstances, the tone of the story and description of the boy's actions does not suggest either of these emotions. The boy is clearly looking forward to the game and is happy that it won't be cancelled due to poor weather.

Questions 17–18: Passage Map

Passage 1: Homework = not fun but useful
Passage 2: Homework = too much time/stressful, probably not useful

17. **(C) They disagree over whether the benefit of completing homework is worth the effort.** It is clear that the first writer is in favor of assigning a lot of homework while the second one is not. The question is why they disagree. Both authors note that completing a large amount of homework is difficult. The first author suggests that this builds character and sets students up for later success. In contrast, the second author suggests that doing a lot of homework is frustrating, interferes with family time, and will not be very useful to the child's future life. So the points of disagreement are whether homework is as beneficial as is claimed and whether any benefits gained are worth the cost. Choice **(C)** is a match for one of these predictions.

18. **(B) A survey of students in kindergarten through grade 12 found that most considered their academic load to be minimal and unchallenging.** There is one thing both authors agree on: homework is difficult. They disagree about whether this is a good thing: one states that homework's difficulty supports a child's development, and the other says it stresses the child out and undermines family time. If the idea that homework is difficult is undermined, then both arguments are weakened. Therefore, choice **(B)** is correct. Choice (A) weakens the first author's argument only, (C) weakens the second author's argument, and (D) is irrelevant to both arguments.

19. **(A) provide a supporting detail for the main idea.** The first sentence introduces the main idea, that "[t]he English language is an amalgam of several other languages, but relies most heavily on Latin." To support this, the author provides an example of an English word that is derived from a Latin prefix and root. Choice **(A)** describes this use of the word "ambidextrous" and is thus correct. Choice (B) is incorrect because the topic is the English language, not this particular word. (C) is incorrect because the paragraph states that we don't translate the word literally from the Latin but instead give it a somewhat different meaning in English. Choice (D) is incorrect because although the root and prefix of "ambidextrous" are Latin, it is an English word.

20. **(A) She is explaining the basis for a marketing decision.** Asafa is laying out the reasons a decision was made by noting the relevance of social media to a marketing campaign. She is not ignoring Janelle as in choice (B); she directly states that the memo answers Janelle's question, and she thanks Janelle for her input. Although the memo begins with the word "Sorry," this relates to a delay in responding, not to any outcome, so choice (C) is incorrect. Finally, Asafa is not suggesting that Janelle use social media, (D).

Questions 21–23: Passage Map

Topic: Astronomy
Scope: Brightness/visibility of objects
Purpose: Explain how improved perception of objects advances astronomy
¶ 1: Moons of Jupiter visible with telescope, proved solar system model; recent technology advanced understanding more
¶ 2: Brightness related to size, distance
Chart: Shows object brightness, higher number means fainter

21. **(D) astronomy has advanced based on our ability to perceive different celestial objects.** This is a main idea question, and the main idea of this passage appears in the first few sentences and is captured in the passage map. Choice **(D)** correctly identifies the main idea, that being able to see relatively faint objects with technology has been key to increasing astronomical knowledge.

22. **(C) the more powerful the telescope, the fainter the objects it can be used to discover.** This inference question does not point to any particular part of the passage, so consult your map and make a mental checklist of the author's key ideas. The correct answer will logically follow from one or more of these. Then check each answer choice against your understanding of the passage. It is noted in the passage that Galileo discovered Jupiter's moons when the telescope became available, and Jupiter's moons are fainter than Earth's own moon (because a higher number means an object is harder to see). These pieces of information strongly imply that telescopes make fainter objects easier to see. The passage also states that the more powerful Hubble telescope allows greater detail to be seen, further supporting the idea that stronger telescopes allow people to see more. None of the other answer choices are supported by the passage.

23. **(A) −26.7** The passage states that brighter objects have a lower apparent magnitude. The brightest object on the table is Earth's moon (Luna), which has a negative value. Because the sun is obviously brighter than the moon, it must have a lower apparent magnitude, that is, less than −12.6. Only one value in the answer choices is less than −12.6—that's −26.7, choice **(A)**.

24. **(C) Some foods taste better when cooked in salted water.** In the last sentence, Chef Marion names pasta as an example of a food that tastes better when cooked in salted water. A statement about which food tastes better reflects the chef's opinion; someone else might think food cooked in unsalted water tastes better. Choice (B) is a scientific fact, not an opinion. Although (A) might be true, Chef Marion does not express an opinion about the healthfulness of foods. You might be tempted by (D), thinking that cooking in hotter water equates to cooking more quickly, but the passage does not support

this idea; it could be that the higher temperature cooks pasta through more thoroughly in the same time, for example.

25. **(A) painting small areas with blue and other colors** Careful reading of both the stimulus and question are vital to getting a correct answer. The question asks for a step that is *not* part of painting a room. There are an infinite number of activities that aren't part of painting a room! Because you can't predict which one will be in the answer choices, check each choice against the passage and eliminate those that are mentioned. The only one not mentioned is choice **(A)**: patches of the wall should be painted different shades of one color (blue is the example used in the passage), not blue and other colors.

Questions 26–27: Passage Map

Topic: Charles Frederick Worth
Scope: Importance as designer, businessperson
Purpose: Argue that he had lasting impact on fashion industry

26. **(C) Its quality of construction and luxuriousness of materials** Worth is described as the "inventor of haute couture," and this is described as establishing new standards for the construction and luxury of clothing. Choice (B) is a detail about the particular customers Worth served, not the clothing he designed. Choice (A) relates to a quality that would not be expected of haute couture; this contrast is signaled by the key word "[d]espite." Nothing in the passage connects choice (D) with haute couture; this is a description of the way the designer ran his business, not his clothing.

27. **(B) Many fashion designers today seek to be well-known among people who cannot afford their clothes.** The author's conclusion, signaled by the key word "[t]hus," is that today's fashion industry has been shaped in part by Worth's passion for self-promotion, which was so great that even women who could not afford his clothes knew who he was. To strengthen the argument, therefore, look for an answer choice that provides further evidence that modern fashion designers are famous beyond their customer base. Choice **(B)** matches this prediction. Choice (A) only reinforces that Worth was important to the history of fashion, not that he had an impact on the contemporary fashion world. Choice (C) is about the lasting impact of his clothing designs, but the author's argument is about the lasting impact of his business model. Whether Worth made money, choice (D), is beside the point, because the author's conclusion is about "superstar" designers—that is, very famous designers, not necessarily rich ones.

28. **(A) Jason had been late to work earlier in the week.** This is an inference question that asks what was *not* implied by the passage. Check each answer choice against what is implied in the story. Because Jason is explaining why he was late,

you can infer that everything he mentions about traffic and detours slowed him down. Thus, he drove down Maple and was affected by the lane closure, as in choice (B). He drives a large truck and couldn't take the faster detour, (D), and due to driving the large truck, he couldn't park in the smaller spaces, (C). Not implied is the idea that he had been late earlier in the week. The passage begins, "What a week it had been!" but that exclamation could refer to any kind of difficulties, not necessarily other days when Jason was late to work.

29. **(D) Problem and solution** The passage states that King George V wanted to recognize the contributions of noncombatants in World War I but was unable to do so and goes on to explain that the MBE was established to solve this deficiency. The passage, therefore, notes a problem and identifies a solution as in choice **(D)**. Choice (A) might have been tempting because the passage discusses a king, the kind of prominent person about whom biographies are often written. However, the focus of the passage is on why the MBE was created and what purpose it serves today; King George V is a supporting detail in that story.

30. **(A) A pooling of hospitals' and clinics' procurement of surgical tools, such as laser scalpels, so these instruments are purchased at lower cost** This inference question requires you to use information from the text and the chart. The author of the passage states that the best opportunities for cost savings lie in the categories that are the biggest percentage of healthcare costs. The pie chart shows that these involve hospitals, choices (B) and (D); physicians and clinics, choice (B); and prescription drugs, choice (C). The passage explains that *nondurable* medical supplies are disposable items, so you can infer that *durable* medical equipment is multiuse items, like surgical tools. At 1%, durable medical equipment is a much smaller category than those involved in the other answer choices, and therefore choice **(A)** is the strategy the author would least likely adopt to achieve cost savings.

31. **(B) It assumes that one daycare worker will be required for each parent who wants to return to work.** The question asks you to identify a problem in the way the letter writer supports her conclusion with evidence. The author's argument is that parents returning to work will not gain financially, because the amount they spend on daycare will almost equal their own daily earnings. However, the argument assumes that each parent will be fully responsible for the wage of a single daycare worker. Common sense suggests that each daycare worker will be responsible for more children than those dropped off by a given parent. For example, if 2 daycare workers are responsible for 20 children of 15 parents, then those parents share the cost of those workers. This is the major flaw in the argument. Choice (A) might be tempting; most parents will need the

daycare worker to take care of the children while the parent is driving to and from work, so the hours that daycare is needed would be more than the hours the parent works. However, this actually strengthens the argument that daycare costs would be too high. Choice (C) is part of the mayor's argument, not the letter writer's. Choice (D) does not describe a flaw in the argument; having a personal opinion on a subject does not invalidate an argument as long as the conclusion proceeds logically from the evidence.

32. **(B) Pleasant** The figure of speech "sunny disposition" is an appropriate way to describe a pleasant person, someone who is always smiling, for example. The other choices all have negative connotations.

33. **(A) Challenging** Martina's choice of words ("waste valuable time") in her response to Thomas reveals that she is challenging his suggestion. Although her first comment is phrased as a question, she is speaking rhetorically and is not really interested in answer, so choice (D), "puzzled," is incorrect. There is nothing "encouraging," (B), or "understanding," (C), in her tone. Indeed, with the words "Everyone knows," Martina is quite dismissive toward Thomas.

Questions 34–38: Passage Map

Topic: Public libraries in America
Scope: Carnegie's support
Purpose: Explain why he supported, positive impact

34. **(C) Public libraries, which are important resources for educating people in a democracy, benefited greatly from Andrew Carnegie's library funding.** To answer this main idea question, it is important to consider the entire passage. Consult your map, where you have jotted notes about the topic, scope, and purpose. Overall, the passage is about Andrew Carnegie's support for public libraries, which are described as being important to "to inform a literate and thoughtful citizenry." The answer that reflects both of these ideas is **(C)**, which summarizes the entire passage. Choice (A) is only about Carnegie, choice (B) is the opposite of the facts in the passage, and choice (D) is only partially correct. Carnegie did believe in free libraries, but nothing in the passage indicates that he believed libraries are the foundation of a thriving democracy.

35. **(A) to serve as an example of Carnegie's support for libraries.** Throughout the passage, the author highlights Carnegie's funding of libraries and his desire to make these sources of knowledge available to all people. The author uses the Washington library as a concrete example of the results of Carnegie's support; the dedication inscribed on the library

provides evidence as to why Carnegie put his money toward public libraries. Choice **(A)** is a match for this prediction. Choices (B) and (D) are out of scope; neither beautification of cities nor access to public buildings in general is mentioned in the passage. Choice (C) reflects the author's viewpoint and does not relate to the use of the Washington library as an example.

36. **(B) Immigrates from Scotland; becomes wealthy; builds the Allegheny library** Research the passage for the progression of events in Carnegie's life. Carnegie is first mentioned at the end of the third sentence. That sentence describes him as a "steel tycoon," and the next sentence describes him as a "self-educated Scottish immigrant." From this, you can infer that he was poor in Scotland, immigrated, and became very wealthy. A few sentences later, the keyword "first" introduces the first library Carnegie build, in Allegheny. This sequence of events matches choice **(B)**. Choice (A) is not only out of order but also out of scope; there is no indication that Carnegie returned to Scotland. Choices (C) and (D) are also out of order.

37. **(D) The very wealthy can afford to downplay the importance of money.** Remember that the correct answer to an inference question, though not stated in the passage, must be true given the information that is stated. The author's parenthetical comment relates to the fact that Carnegie had become a very wealthy man by being a "ruthless businessman" and keeping the wages of his workers down, yet said he prioritized knowledge over money. The author is commenting on the fact that someone with no need to focus on financial security has the luxury of valuing knowledge, and the author extends this insight to wealthy people in general. Thus, the correct answer is choice **(D)**. Choice (A) reflects Carnegie's expressed viewpoint but not the author's. Choices (B) and (C) misrepresent the author's point; the author does not judge Carnegie's stated belief in the importance of knowledge.

38. **(B) They provide needed information for knowledgeable citizens.** In the first sentence, the author states that libraries were prized. She goes on to write that "they were deemed important sources of knowledge to inform a literate and thoughtful citizenry." Though choice **(B)** states this in different words, it is a match for what the author writes in the passage. Choice (A) is stated in the passage but is a relatively minor detail. Choice (D) is also true according to the passage, but this is a description of how libraries work, not why they are fundamentally important. Choice (C) is contradicted by the passage; the author states that libraries are often funded by taxes, but as Carnegie's library building efforts make clear, this was not always the case. Be careful of answer choices with the extreme word "always," because they are only correct if the author uses equally extreme language.

Questions 39–40: Passage Map

Topic: Pro cycling "Grand Tour"
Scope: The three races
Purpose: Inform reader of some history

39. **(B) The second sentence** In the second sentence, the author expresses the opinion that the Tour de France is the "most enjoyable" of the Grand Tour races. The first sentence states a fact, and the fourth sentence reflects a value judgment ("most prestigious") made by other people, not the author.

40. **(B) Giro d'Italia, Tour de France, Vuelta a España** Correctly answering this detail question requires careful reading of the passage. You are told that the Tour de France is usually held in July. You are also told that the Vuelta a España was "originally run in April, not long before the Giro d'Italia," which means the latter race is held shortly after April. Now, you are told, the Vuelta a España takes place in the fall. So, the current running order of the Grand Tour is the Giro d'Italia (sometime shortly after April), the Tour de France (usually in July), and the Vuelta a España (sometime in the fall). Note that choice (A) is the order in which the races were first run, but this is not what the question is asking for.

41. **(C) Sadly** This is the meaning of "dolefully." If you weren't sure of the word's meaning, the sentence provides clues. The contrasting word "but" means Marcus was feeling the opposite of "happy." Therefore, you can infer that "dolefully" is similar in meaning to "sadly." Choice (D), "warily," also has a negative connotation, but it means "being worried about potential danger," and there is no reason to think Marcus was afraid of his future wife, only that he was not happy for some reason.

Questions 42–43: Passage Map

Topic: Mining in space
Scope: The "old man's" foolish optimism
Purpose: To tell a story, describing a setting and lifestyle
In these ¶s, two men discuss a miner who is losing money while hoping to strike it rich; Buck and Cole poke fun at the "old man's" dreams.

42. **(A) Miners are practical in the everyday details of their work but have wildly optimistic dreams of making their fortune.** This question asks for the overall theme of the two characters' dialogue, in which the character of a miner, the "old man," is made clear through the viewpoint of Buck and Cole. The correct answer will express their characterization of the miner. The miner spends 101% of his output, that is, 1% more than he makes; thus, he is slowly losing money. It's then explained that he is operating at maximum efficiency in the

sense of making his losses as small as possible. When Buck asks about the miner's motives, Cole clarifies that he wants to get rich and retire. So his goal is to make his money last as long as possible in hopes of striking it rich, a goal the two characters view with skepticism. Finally, Cole says "all" miners have this dream. Thus, the miner is both shrewd in managing his operation and foolish in envisioning his future. Choice **(A)** expresses the overall gist of the passage. The other choices are either contradicted by the passage or express only part of its meaning.

43. **(C) jovium is both rarer and more valuable than platinum.** Because this is an inference question, the correct answer choice will be something that follows from statements in the passage, and the other answer choices will be either untrue or not necessarily true. The passage states that the miner has a "rich" platinum mine but is losing money, meaning there is a lot of the metal but it is not worth enough to cover the cost of mining it. The fact that the miner hasn't found jovium yet indicates that it is rarer than platinum, and the fact that he expects to retire if he does find jovium means it is more valuable. Beyond what you know from the passage itself, it is common knowledge that rare things tend to be more valuable than common things, so when you infer one, you can reasonably infer the other. None of the other statements can be inferred from the passage. Choice (A) is extreme; there isn't enough information here to know what eventually happens to most miners. Choice (B) is not supported: Buck and Cole poke fun at the miners, but they do not express a negative opinion or view themselves as better than the miners. Choice (D): While Buck and Cole appear to be friendly, they may have been friends for years without working together, or they may have become friendly quickly.

44. **(A) Military training helps build "grit."** The author is arguing that children without grit get less from their education, and that expensive schools are therefore a waste. He argues that these children should go to boot camp instead of prep school. The assumption is that boot camp will help them build character, or "grit." Choice (B) is the opposite of what the author believes, as is (C), because the point of grit is to do more work and learn more. Choice (D) might be tempting, but the author only suggests that lazy children are sent to expensive schools, not that sending the kids to those schools actually makes them lazy.

45. **(D) Buy a photo postcard of Edinburgh Castle.** The writer states that Naresh advised a trip to Edinburgh, (C); talked the writer into buying hiking boots, (B); and told him to bring an umbrella, (A). On the other hand, he writes that he is surprising Naresh with this postcard, so **(D)** is the correct choice.

46. **(A) Is Edinburgh a beautiful city?** Naresh advised the writer to "go someplace beautiful." Using Naresh's opinion as evidence, the writer concluded that he should go to Edinburgh. To move from this evidence to this conclusion, the writer must have determined that Edinburgh is beautiful by asking the question in choice **(A)**. The postcard writer decided to visit Edinburgh despite being told by Naresh that it was expensive, so evaluating whether Edinburgh was more or less expensive than other places was not essential to reaching the decision to go there. Choice (D) is incorrect.

47. **(D) "I make sure my watch battery is charged."** The author states that she sets her alarm before a workday only after she ensures her watch battery is charged. The other two steps take place when she wakes the next day.

Questions 48–49: Passage Map

Topic: News reporting
Scope: Inaccuracy, bias
Purpose: To criticize

48. **(D) illustrate ways in which the media depart from unbiased news reporting.** Throughout, the author contrasts an ideal of unbiased news coverage with the biased reporting that actually occurs. Graphics and sound effects are mentioned in the second sentence, where according to the author they are used to "entice viewers and garner ratings." The next sentence continues: "Real facts . . . are totally abandoned." Thus, graphics and sound effects are examples of what the media does to make a story interesting, which, in turn, leads to inaccuracy and bias. Choice **(D)** is a match for this prediction. Choice (A) is true in that the graphics and sound effects are designed to make the story interesting, but relevance is not mentioned in the passage. Furthermore, the author presents these examples to say something negative about the news media, not something positive. The author considers biased news "junk," not the graphics and sound effects that are features of that news, as in choice (B). Similarly, the author does distinguish two kinds of reporting, but not solely on the basis of graphics and sound effects, (C); the distinction lies in accuracy and bias.

49. **(D) condemn the media for distorting news reports.** From the very first sentence, the author severely criticizes the news media for abandoning "[r]eal facts and unbiased coverage of an issue . . . in exchange for an overly sentimental or one-sided story that too often distorts the truth." Choice **(D)**, which uses the strong word "condemn," meaning to express strong disapproval, reflects this purpose. Choice (A) might be tempting, but the author isn't criticizing viewers; instead, she is warning them of the dangers of distorted news reports. (B) is

the opposite of the author's point. The author does distinguish between biased and neutral reporting, but simply explaining the difference is not her primary purpose, (C).

Questions 50–51: Passage Map

Topic: Minors workings on family farms
Scope: License requirements to operate heavy equipment
Purpose: The first passage explains the goal of the bill. The second passage argues against it.
Passage 1: News article; kids age 14 1/2 up need license to operate tractors
Passage 2: Law will hurt farming families; parents know better than government how to run business, raise kids

50. **(B) The farmer disagrees with the state senators' assumptions about safety issues in child farm labor.** The argument of the state officials, as described in the news article, is that restricting minors' access to farm equipment will make those children safer. The farmer argues that this law will make farmers' lives more difficult and that the officials know little about how to keep children safe on farms. The key disagreement, then, is about whether the senators understand the safety concerns at issue, answer choice **(B)**. Choice (A) is out of scope because the debate is about children on farms operating heavy equipment, not children doing any kind of work. Choice (C) is incorrect as neither party compares safety and economic security. Choice (D) is incorrect: the senate has passed a law restricting the operation of heavy equipment, not farmwork in general, and the farmer claims "we've always taken good care of our kids," meaning that farmwork poses little risk.

51. **(D) the state overestimates the danger to children of operating tractors.** The word "apparently" indicates that this is an inference question, so the correct answer choice will include an idea believed by the second author but not explicitly stated. The crux of the second author's argument is that this bill makes farm families' lives more difficult without improving safety, because farmers know better than legislators how to raise their children safely, choice **(D)**. He does not imply that safety is not important, choice (C), nor does he imply that the state is intentionally trying to hurt the agriculture industry, (B). Indeed, he implies they are hurting the industry due to ignorance. There's no reference to hiring children to work on land not owned by their family, so choice (A) is irrelevant.

52. **(A) while** The author states that three species of frigate birds are widespread but two are endangered with restricted breeding habitats, so look for a word that signals contrast. Choice **(A)**, "while," matches the prediction.

53. **(D) constructive** This word means "helping to improve." Choice (A), "shift," is neutral, simply meaning "a change." The words "pejorative" ("belittling") and "vilification" ("harsh criticism") have negative meanings. If you weren't sure of the words' meanings, you could use context clues to find the answer. The word "Fortunately" indicates that the campaign has changed in a positive manner. Thus, it has changed "from [a bad thing] to [a good thing]," and the latter phrase will contain the word with a positive connotation.

Mathematics

1. **(B) 0.045** This question asks you to convert a percent to a decimal. You may have memorized the very useful shortcut "Move the decimal two places to the left and drop the % sign." This will efficiently produce the correct answer to this straightforward question. However, be sure to understand the process as well. Convert the percentage to a fraction by placing the expression over 100 and then change the fraction to a decimal by using place value: $4.5\% = \frac{4.5}{100} = \frac{4.5(10)}{100(10)} = \frac{45}{1000} = 0.045$.

2. **(A) Skewed right** The question presents a bar graph and asks for a description of the distribution indicated by the shape of the graph. *Skew* describes the direction of the "tail" of a graph (i.e., the part of the graph with fewer data values). Because this graph's tail is to the right, the graph indicates a distribution that is skewed right.

3. **(A) 23** The question provides an equation with a variable on one side and a value on the other, and it requires you to isolate the variable. Use inverse operations to isolate y. First, subtract 36 from both sides to yield $4y = 92$. Next, divide both sides by 4 to yield $y = 23$.

4. **(D) 360** The question provides the rate at which the worker slices oranges and the number of slices per orange, and it asks for the number of slices the worker will produce in 15 minutes. First, calculate how many oranges the worker can cut up in one minute: $\frac{60 \text{ seconds per minute}}{15 \text{ seconds per orange}} = 4$ oranges per minute. Next, calculate how many oranges he can cut up in 15 minutes: 4 oranges per minute × 15 minutes = 60 oranges in 15 minutes. Finally, calculate the number of slices: 60 oranges × 6 slices = 360 slices.

5. **(A) There was a positive covariance between the number of telephones and the incidence of cancer.** You are provided survey data: the more telephones in a household, the more likely it was that a member of the household had cancer. Then

the question asks which of the answer choices best describes the relationship between those two variables. Based on the limited information given, all you can conclude is that there is a positive relationship between telephones and cancer. This positive relationship is a covariance between the two measurements, so choice (A) is correct. Choice (B) is the opposite. Choice (D) says that there is a cause-and-effect relationship (that talking on the phone causes cancer), and choice (C) says that there is no cause and effect involved. A common error in logic is to assume that a correlation between two things means that a cause-and-effect relationship exists. There is not enough information here to know whether there is or is not a causal relationship between telephones and cancer, so both (C) and (D) are incorrect.

6. **(C) 29** The question provides the part-to-part ratio of three of the four colors of marbles in a bag (red, white, and blue). It also states that there are half as many green marbles as there are blue marbles. You need to find the minimum total number of marbles that satisfies these facts. Because the number of green marbles is half that of blue marbles, restate the part-to-part ratio by adding green at the end. The number in the ratio representing blue is 5, so the number representing green is half that, or $2\frac{1}{2}$. Thus, the ratio becomes $3:4:5:2\frac{1}{2}$.

However, there won't be half a marble, so double all the values to get 6:8:10:5. While the total number of marbles could be the sum of the values in the part-to-part ratio multiplied by any number, the question asks for the *least* possible number, so just add $6 + 8 + 10 + 5$ to get 29, choice **(C)**.

7. **(C) 135** The pie chart provides the percentages of apple trees of different ages, and the question tells you the total number of trees. You need to find the number of trees 5 years old or younger. Find the segments of the chart that include ages of 5 years or younger. The chart indicates that 20% of the trees are less than 3 years old and 25% are from 3 to 5 years old, so add these two percentages: $20\% + 25\% = 45\%$. Now calculate 45% of the total number of trees: $0.45 \times 300 = 135$.

8. **(D)** $\frac{1}{2}$ The question provides the total number of eggs and the number of eggs painted each color other than green, and it asks for the fraction of eggs that are painted green. Begin by determining the number of eggs that are painted a color other than green: 5 blue + 5 yellow + 5 pink = 15 eggs that are not green. Subtract this number from the total number of eggs to calculate the number that are green: 30 total eggs − 15 eggs that are not green = 15 green eggs. Thus, the fraction of green

eggs to total eggs is $\frac{15}{30}$. Because this fraction does not appear among the answer choices, simplify: $\frac{15}{30} = \frac{1}{2}$.

9. **(A) 2,399,679** The question asks for the product of four 2-digit numbers. The answer choices are closely spaced, so estimating will not suffice. Rather than accessing the calculator, however, look at the last digits of the four numbers. The last digit of the product of $27 \times 47 \times 31 \times 61$ is the same as the last digit of $7 \times 7 \times 1 \times 1 = 49$—the last digit is 9. The only answer choice that ends in 9 is **(A)**. This shortcut doesn't always work because there could be more than one answer choice that ends in the target number. However, it is so fast and simple that it is always worth a try, especially in a case like this where every answer choice ends with a different digit.

10. **(D) 6** You are asked to multiply two mixed numbers. Change each number to an improper fraction: $1\frac{7}{8} \times 3\frac{1}{5} = \frac{15}{8} \times \frac{16}{5}$. Simplify before multiplying if possible by dividing out common factors from the numerator and denominator: $\frac{15 \times 16}{8 \times 5} = \frac{3 \times 2}{1 \times 1}$. Now multiply the numerators and then the denominators: $\frac{6}{1} = 6$.

11. **(C) 5 decimeters** A wide elastic band requires 40 g weight of force to stretch it 1 mm. The force-to-distance relationship is linear, so each additional millimeter of stretch will add 40 grams of resistance. The maximum force permitted is 20 kg. The question asks how far the band can stretch to produce that much force. The information in the question is in different metric units, and the answer choices are presented in various metric units as well, so conversion of units will be part of solving this question. Begin by converting 20 kg to 20,000 g. Then, to determine the distance that would create that much force, divide 20,000 g by 40 g/mm to get 500 mm. Choice (A), 5 mm, is clearly incorrect. None of the other answer choices are stated in mm. Since there are 10 mm per cm, 500 mm = 50 cm, so (B) is incorrect as well. There are 10 cm per decimeter, so 50 cm = 5 decimeters and choice **(C)** is correct.

12. **(A) 36 − 9π** The question provides a circle inscribed in a square, and it asks you to find the area of that region of the square not bounded by the circle. Find the area of each shape and then subtract the area of the circle from the area of the square. The area of a square is side length squared: $6^2 = 36$ square inches. Because the side length of the square is 6 inches, this must also be the diameter of the circle. The area formula for a circle is πr^2. Because the diameter is 6 inches, the radius is 3 inches, so the area of the circle is $\pi 3^2 = 9\pi$ square inches. Thus, the area of the shaded region is $36 − 9\pi$ square inches.

13. **(B)** $\frac{13}{4}$, **3.35,** $\frac{7}{2}$, $\frac{11}{3}$, **4** You are asked to order the numbers from least to greatest. Given the mix of fractions and decimals, it may be easiest to convert the fractions to decimals: $\frac{11}{3} = 3.\overline{66}$, $\frac{13}{4} = 3.25$, $\frac{7}{2} = 3.5$. Now compare the numbers:
$\frac{13}{4} < 3.35 < \frac{7}{2} < \frac{11}{3} < 4$.

14. **(B) $16 \leq n \leq 48$** The question provides the minimum and maximum number of times the nurse will record the client's blood pressure each hour and the duration of the shift in hours, and it asks for the expression that reflects the number of times the blood pressure will be recorded. To calculate the range of the possible number of times n the nurse will record blood pressure over the entire shift, multiply the minimum number of times per hour and the maximum number of times per hour by the number of hours in the shift: minimum: 2 times per hour × 8 hours = 16 times; maximum: 6 times per hour × 8 hours = 48 times. Thus, n is greater than or equal to 16, and less than or equal to 48.

15. **(B) 4** The question provides the sports drink's concentration level, the amount of nutrient mix in each bottle, and the total amount of sports drink the trainer will produce. You need to determine how many total bottles of nutrient mix the trainer will need. Determine the quantity of the nutrient mix needed by multiplying the amount of sports drink by the concentrate level: 15% of 240 ounces = 0.15 × 240 ounces = 36 ounces of nutrient mix. Next, determine how many bottles of nutrient mix the trainer will need to purchase by dividing the total amount of mix needed by the amount of mix per bottle: 36 ounces of nutrient mix ÷ 10 ounces per bottle = 3.6 bottles. Because the trainer has to purchase the nutrient mix by the bottle, she'll need to buy 4 bottles.

16. **(D)** $2\frac{11}{24}$ To add fractions with different denominators, you first need a to find common denominator. The least common denominator (LCD) of these fractions is 24. Using 24 as the denominator, rewrite each fraction:
$\frac{7}{8} + \frac{5}{6} + \frac{3}{4} = \frac{7 \times 3}{8 \times 3} + \frac{5 \times 4}{6 \times 4} + \frac{3 \times 6}{4 \times 6} = \frac{21}{24} + \frac{20}{24} + \frac{18}{24}$. Add the numerators of the fractions: $\frac{21 + 20 + 18}{24} = \frac{59}{24}$. Simplify the fraction: $2\frac{11}{24}$.

17. **(A)** $\frac{4}{15}$ The question provides values for the ratios of a to b and b to c and asks for the ratio of a to c. To work with these ratios, translate them into their fractional representations:

$\frac{a}{b} = \frac{4}{3}$ and $\frac{b}{c} = \frac{1}{5}$. The ratio $\frac{a}{c}$ can be calculated by multiplying the two known ratios: $\frac{a}{b} \times \frac{b}{c} = \frac{a}{c}$. Substitute the known values for those ratios to get $\frac{4}{3} \times \frac{1}{5} = \frac{4}{15}$, which is choice **(A)**.

18. **(D) 20** The graph shows the number of households that own zero, one, two, three, or four cars. The question asks you to determine how many households own three or more cars. The graph indicates that 15 households own three cars and five households own four cars. Add these together: 15 households + 5 households = 20 households.

19. **(C) 118** The question asks for the value of an expression "to the nearest whole number," which, along with the wide spacing of the answer choices, is a clue that estimating would be a good approach. Round 31 down to 30 and roll 917 down to 900. Now simply solve 900 ÷ 30 × 4 = 30 × 4 = 120. The only answer choice close to that estimate is **(C)**. Although you have access to a calculator on the TEAS, in this case, estimating is probably just as quick and avoids the risk of data entry errors.

20. **(B) 864 L** The question states that a tank contains 180 L + 360 L = 540 L and that it is $\frac{5}{8}$ full. You must find the total capacity of the tank. Set up the proportion $\frac{540}{C} = \frac{5}{8}$. Cross multiply to get $8 \times 540 = 5C$. Simplify the calculations by first dividing both sides by 5: $8 \times 108 = C$; $864 = C$. Answer choice **(B)** is correct.

21. **(A) 2,000,000** The question provides an amount in kilograms and asks for a conversion from kilograms to milligrams. Use dimensional analysis (the fact that multiplying or dividing a value by 1 does not change the value) to convert from kilograms to milligrams: 2 kilograms × $\frac{1,000 \text{ grams}}{1 \text{ kilogram}}$ × $\frac{1,000 \text{ milligrams}}{1 \text{ gram}}$ = 2,000,000 milligrams.

22. **(C) $q = p + 4$** The question asks you to determine which of the equations in the answer choices results in a positive covariance between the two variables. Choice (A) may be tempting, but because q is a function of p squared, p can become a smaller and smaller negative number yet q will continue to get larger. Eliminate (A). The equation in (B) simplifies to $q = 4$, so there is no relationship with p. In **(C)**, as p increases, so does q, so the two variables are positively covariant. In choice (D), as p increases, q decreases, so the two are negatively covariant.

23. **(B) $9a - 15$** The question presents an algebraic expression containing a single variable and asks you to find the equivalent expression among the answer choices. Simplify and combine like terms to isolate the variable a. First, simplify the fraction by dividing the numerator by 2 to yield $2(a - 8)$. Next, distribute the 2 to get $2a - 16$. Now combine like terms: $6a + 2a + a = 9a$ and $-16 + 1 = -15$. Finally, add the resulting terms: $9a + (-15) = 9a - 15$. Note that another way to solve would be to substitute a number for a. If $a = 2$, then the expression equals $(6)(2) + \dfrac{4(2-8)}{2} + 2 + 1 = 3$. Plugging in 2 for a in each of the answer choices produces 3 only in choice **(B)**.

24. **(B) 45 miles** The question provides the number of segments of a trip, the bicyclist's speed for each segment of the trip, and the time it takes to cover the first two segments, as well as the time for the entire trip. You are asked to determine the entire distance. Use the formula rate $\times$ time $=$ distance. First, calculate the distance of the uphill segment: 20 minutes $\times$ 15 mph $= \dfrac{1}{3}$ hour $\times$ 15 mph $=$ 5 miles. Next, the level segment: 1 hour $\times$ 20 mph $=$ 20 miles. To find the distance of the downhill segment, first calculate the time it takes to travel this segment by subtracting the time of the other two segments from the entire trip length: 2 hours $-$ 1 hour 20 minutes $=$ 40 minutes. Next, calculate the distance: 40 minutes $\times$ 30 mph $= \dfrac{2}{3}$ hour $\times$ 30 mph $=$ 20 miles. Finally, add all three distances: 5 miles $+$ 20 miles $+$ 20 miles $=$ 45 miles.

25. **(B) 19.5%** The question provides a price before sales tax, the sales tax rate, and the total amount including a tip. You are asked what percentage of the price plus tax was the tip. A key element of this question is the amount of the meal plus tax. Apply the 6% tax rate to the base amount: $\dfrac{6}{100} \times 110.50 = 0.06 \times 110.50 = \$6.63$. Add this tax to the amount for food and beverages: $\$110.50 + \$6.63 = \$117.13$. Because the total charge was \$140, the amount of the gratuity must have been $\$140 - \$117.13 = \$22.87$. Calculate the percent tip relative to the bill with tax added: $\dfrac{t}{100} = \dfrac{22.87}{117.13}$. Cross multiply to get $117.13t = 2287$. Divide both sides of the equation by 117.13 to get $t = 19.5\%$, which is choice **(B)**. Choice (C) is the tip amount as a percentage of the bill *before* tax, and choice (D) ignores tax altogether.

26. **(B) 155** You are asked the value of an expression with multiple operations. The order of operations is important. Use PEMDAS. Start inside the parentheses, doing multiplication/division first and then addition/

subtraction: $2 \times (80 - 5) + 5 = 2 \times (75) + 5$. Next, multiply: $2 \times 75 + 5 = 150 + 5$. Last, add: $150 + 5 = 155$.

27. **(D) 1:6** The question provides the total area of the garden, the number of carrot seeds planted per square foot, the number of lettuce seeds planted per square foot, and the fraction of the garden's area planted with carrot seeds. You need to solve for the ratio of lettuce seeds to carrot seeds. Begin by calculating the number of square feet planted in carrots: $\dfrac{2}{3} \times 60$ square feet $=$ 40 square feet. Multiply this by the number of carrot seeds per square foot: 40 square feet $\times$ 6 carrot seeds $=$ 240 carrot seeds total. Next, calculate the remaining square footage: 60 total square feet $-$ 40 square feet planted with carrot seeds $=$ 20 square feet planted with lettuce seeds. Multiply this number by the number of lettuce seeds per square foot: 20 square feet $\times$ 2 lettuce seeds $=$ 40 lettuce seeds total. Finally, set up the ratio of lettuce seeds to carrot seeds and simplify: $40:240 = 1:6$. Make sure you have the ratio of lettuce to carrot seeds and not the other way around.

28. **(C) -53%** The question provides the fractional contents of a bottle of water at two different times and asks for the percentage change of the contents between those times. Note that the first measurement is that $\dfrac{2}{7}$ of the water had been *consumed*, which means that $\dfrac{5}{7}$ remained. The percentage change is the second observed amount less the first amount divided by the first amount and converted to percent, or $\dfrac{\dfrac{1}{3} - \dfrac{5}{7}}{\dfrac{5}{7}} \times 100\%$.

Multiply every term by 21 to eliminate the fractions:

$$\dfrac{21\left(\dfrac{1}{3}\right) - 21\left(\dfrac{5}{7}\right)}{21\left(\dfrac{5}{7}\right)} \times 100\% = \dfrac{7 - 15}{15} \times 100\%.$$

This equals -53% to the nearest percent, so choice **(C)** is correct. Note that because water is consumed and no water is added $\left(\dfrac{1}{3} < \dfrac{5}{7}\right)$, the percentage change must be negative.

Thus, you could eliminate choices (A) and (B) on that basis alone.

29. **(B) 20** The graph shows the number of clinics in four regions for the years 1950 and 2000. The question asks for the average of the number of clinics in two of the regions in 1950. Find the number in each region in 1950 (the white bars), then calculate their average. In the South, the number of clinics in 1950 was 10; in the West, the number of clinics in

1950 was 30. Apply the average formula: sum of terms divided by number of terms: $\frac{10+30}{2} = \frac{40}{2} = 20$.

30. **(D) 99** The question states that the ratio of two quantities is 7:2 and that if the amount of the first item were increased by 6, the new ratio would be 11:4. You need to solve for the original total number of the two items. The ratio 7:2 gives the relative amounts of brand-name and generic medicine, but the actual amounts could be any multiple of the ratio, so express this as $\frac{7x}{2x}$. When 6 more containers of the generic medicine are added, the quantity of that item is $2x + 6$. The ratio of the new amounts is 11:4, so set up the proportion $\frac{7x}{2x+6} = \frac{11}{4}$. Cross multiply to get $28x = 22x + 66$, so $6x = 66$ and $x = 11$. This is not the answer to the question; it is the multiplier for the initial ratio. The total number of items before the extra 6 were added was $7x + 2x = 9x$. Because $x = 11$, there were 99 containers.

31. **(B) 16** You are asked for the value of an expression with multiple operations. The order of operations is important. Use PEMDAS. Start inside the parentheses:

$3 + 5 \times (8 + 4) \div 3 - 7 = 3 + 5 \times (12) \div 3 - 7$. Next, multiply and divide, from left to right:

$3 + 5 \times 12 \div 3 - 7 = 3 + 60 \div 3 - 7 = 3 + 20 - 7$. Finally, add and subtract, from left to right: $3 + 20 - 7 = 23 - 7 = 16$.

32. **(C) 50** The question provides an equation with the same variable on each side, and it asks you to solve for the variable. Use inverse operations to isolate m. First, add 15 to both sides to yield $3m = \frac{m}{2} + 125$. Next, subtract $\frac{m}{2}$ from both sides to yield $3m - \frac{m}{2} = 125$. To make calculations easier, multiply each term by 2 to eliminate the fraction: $(2)3m - (2)\frac{m}{2} = (2)125$; $6m - m = 250$. Simplify on the left to yield $5m = 250$. Now divide both sides by 5 to yield $m = 50$.

33. **(C) 49** The question provides a diagram of a rectangle with its dimensions, and it asks you to determine the area of a square that has the same perimeter as the rectangle. Begin by determining the perimeter of the rectangle. Perimeter of a rectangle is two times length plus two times width: $(2 \times 9) + (2 \times 5) = 18 + 10 = 28$. Because this is the perimeter of the rectangle, it is also the perimeter of the square. The area of a square is side times side, so you'll need to determine the side length of the square to calculate its area. The perimeter of a square is four times its side length. Therefore, you can find side length by dividing perimeter by four: $28 \div 4 = 7$. Now multiply this length times itself to find the area of the square: $7 \times 7 = 49$.

34. **(B) 39,000 bushels** The graph displays yearly production of sorghum, and you are asked for the production in 2015. No value is shown for 2015, but the question states that 2015 production was half that of 2012. First, estimate the 2012 production from the graph; it was approximately 80,000 bushels. Half that would be 40,000 bushels. However, a closer look at the column for 2012 production shows that it is a couple thousand *less* than 80,000 bushels. This makes choice **(B)**, 39,000 bushels, correct. Choice (A), 36,000, is half the production of 2010, and choice (D) is half that of 2013.

35. **(A) 140.8** The question provides an amount in kilograms and asks for a conversion to an amount in ounces. Use dimensional analysis (the fact that multiplying or dividing a value by 1 does not change the value) to convert kilograms to ounces:

$$4 \text{ kilograms} \times \frac{2.2 \text{ pounds}}{1 \text{ kilogram}} \times \frac{16 \text{ ounces}}{1 \text{ pound}} = 140.8.$$

36. **(D) 88 feet** The question provides the shapes and dimensions of two enclosures and asks for the total length of fencing needed to enclose each completely. To calculate the total length of fencing needed, calculate the perimeter of each of the enclosures separately and then combine the two values. The perimeter of a square is four times the side length, so the kennel's perimeter is 4×9 feet $= 36$ feet. The perimeter of a rectangle is two times length plus two times width, so the dog run is $(2 \times 20 \text{ feet}) + (2 \times 6 \text{ feet}) = 52$ feet. Add the two perimeters: 36 feet + 52 feet = 88 feet.

Science

1. **(C) Dendrites, axon, and soma** The question asks about parts of the neuron. Recall that soma, nucleus, axon, and dendrites are parts of a neuron. The correct answer will contain some or all of these terms and not any others. Choice **(C)** is a match. Choice (A) describes parts of the nervous system, whereas choices (B) and (D) are divisions of the nervous system.

2. **(C) Mitochondrion** This question is asking you for an organelle that is *not* involved in protein production. Recall that mitochondria are responsible for energy production and are not involved in protein production. The ribosome and the rough ER, choices (A) and (B) respectively, are responsible for protein translation. The Golgi apparatus, (D), is involved in protein modification.

3. **(D) Vitamin B$_{12}$** This question is asking about absorption specific to the ileum, the third part of the small intestine, so eliminate any substance that is absorbed elsewhere in the digestive tract. Vitamin K, (A), is absorbed throughout the intestinal tract, not primarily in the ileum. Carbohydrates, (B), are primarily absorbed in the jejunum, another part of the small intestine. Water, (C), is absorbed in the stomach and large intestine.

4. **(A) hypodermis, dermis, epidermis** This question is asking about the layers of the skin. Recall that the skin has three layers: hypodermis, dermis, and epidermis. The dermis is the middle layer that contains the sebaceous glands (which appear in choices (B) and (C)). The lower layer is the hypodermis, and the surface layer is the epidermis. This matches answer choice **(A)**.

5. **(A) 2 and d** This question is asking for a pairing that is *not* possible. Recall that the period number will limit the possible orbitals. In period 2, the only possible orbital names are *s* and *p*, so choices (C) and (D) can be eliminated because they are possible. By the same logic, you can choose choice **(A)**, because orbital *d* cannot appear with period 2. In period number 3, the possible orbital names are *s*, *p*, and *d*, so (B) is a possible pairing and can be eliminated.

6. **(B) Hemoglobin not properly binding to oxygen** This question is asking which factor is *not* a secondary effect of hypertension. Recall that *hypertension* is a term for chronic high blood pressure. Thus, you can eliminate all answer choices that could result from increased pressure in the blood vessels. Minor tearing to the blood vessels can result from the increased pressure, which in turn would cause scar tissue to accumulate, as in choice (A). Vascular scarring can act like a net to catch other particles in the circulatory system, including platelets and cholesterol, causing clots to form. These can both decrease blood flow to vital organs by restricting blood flow, as in choice (D), or can break off and result in a stroke, (C). Choice **(B)** is correct. Poor oxygenation resulting from hypertension is caused by blocked blood vessels, not improper hemoglobin binding.

7. **(D) Storing urea** This question is asking for a role the kidneys do *not* perform, so three of the answer choices will correctly state the kidneys' function. Recall that the kidneys filter blood to remove waste products, choice (A), and they reabsorb water to stabilize blood pressure, (B). The kidneys also convert vitamin D to its active form, as in choice (C). While the kidneys filter urea from the blood, urea (in the form of urine) is stored in the bladder prior to excretion. The correct answer is choice **(D)**.

8. **(C) 10,000 mg** This question is asking for a unit conversion. Recall that 1 gram is equal to 1000 milligrams, so 10 grams must be equal to $10 \times 1000 = 10,000$ milligrams.

9. **(A) Aorta** This question is asking about the variance of blood pressure over different parts of the circulatory system. Recall that blood pressure is highest as it leaves the heart, so predict that the correct answer will be a large artery. This matches choice **(A)**. Though blood is also being pumped directly from the right ventricle to pulmonary arteries, choice (C), the left ventricle is pumping blood through the aorta to the entire body and thus pumps with more force. Blood pressure is lowest in the capillaries, choice (B), and the vena cava, (D), is part of the venous system.

10. **(A) a** The question is asking you to match an endocrine process to the proper endocrine gland. Recall that melatonin is the hormone that regulates sleep, and it is secreted by the pineal gland. The pineal gland is indicated by letter *a* on the diagram. Letter *d* refers to the thyroid gland, which regulates metabolism; *f* to the thymus, which produces T-cells; and *g* to the adrenal glands, which regulate blood pressure as well as release estrogen, androgens, epinephrine, and cortisol, among other secretions.

11. **(B) c** Given the glands and organs represented in the diagram, this question is asking about communication within the endocrine system. Recall that most endocrine organs receive and relay chemical signals in the form of hormones. The exception to this is *c*, which refers to the hypothalamus. The hypothalamus receives electrical impulses from the brain. The label *b* refers to the pituitary gland, which is stimulated by one of several hypothalamic hormones; *e* refers to the parathyroid glands, which are stimulated chemically by calcium; and *k* refers to the ovaries, which are stimulated by LH or FSH.

12. **(C) k** This question is asking about the relationship between luteinizing hormone (LH) and progesterone. Recall that LH is released from the pituitary gland, labeled *b* on the diagram. In males, it stimulates the production of testosterone in the testes, labeled *m*. In females, it stimulates ovulation. After ovulation, the follicle develops into the corpus luteum, which secretes progesterone. This occurs in the ovaries, labeled *k*. The label *j* refers to the uterus.

13. **(C) Decrease gas exchange** This question is asking for a function that surfactant does *not* perform. Recall that surfactant decreases surface tension to prevent lung collapse and serves as a medium for gas exchange. Thus, answer choices (A), (B), and (D) can be eliminated. Surfactant does not decrease gas exchange, so choice **(C)** is correct.

14. **(C) Gastrin stimulates the release of HCl and pepsinogen.** This question is asking about chemical digestion in the stomach. Recall that the stomach secretes two main hormones (gastrin and ghrelin) and three main enzymes (gastric lipase, pepsinogen, and HCl). Gastrin stimulates the release of HCl and pepsinogen, which is converted to pepsin in the presence of acid. This matches choice **(C)**. Gherlin, choice (B), stimulates the appetite, not the exocrine cells of the stomach. Goblet cells, (D), are present in the stomach, but they release mucus. Glucagon, (A), is secreted by the pancreas.

15. **(A) Neurotransmitters** The question is asking what occurs at the synapse between a motor neuron and muscle fiber. Recall that neurotransmitters, such as acetylcholine, are released from the motor neuron and transmit the motor impulse to the muscles. Choice **(A)** is correct. After the neurotransmitters bind to the muscle fibers, calcium ions, (C), are released. The nodes of Ranvier, (B), are gaps in the axon's myelin sheath, and action potentials, (D), propel the motor impulse along the neuron.

16. **(A) Sweat gland activity and blood flow to the subcutaneous layer of the skin increase, and hair follicles relax.** This question is asking about thermoregulation. Recall that one of the primary roles of the integumentary system is to maintain internal body temperature. Sweat glands lower the body temperature via evaporative cooling. Blood vessels dilate to increase heat loss by convection and conduction. Hair follicles relax, causing hairs to lie flat on the skin's surface to prevent heat from becoming trapped against the skin. This response to increased body temperature matches answer choice **(A)**.

17. **(B) Renin** This question is asking about the enzymatic regulation of blood pressure in arteries. Recall that blood pressure can be controlled by vasodilation or vasoconstriction of the blood vessels and by changes to the volume of water that is excreted or reabsorbed by the kidneys, so predict that the correct answer affects one of these processes. Choice **(B)** matches your prediction. Renin is a renal enzyme that activates hormones responsible for regulating blood pressure and fluid balance. Epinephrine, choice (A), is a hormone that causes vasodilation or constriction; however, the question specifically asks for an enzyme. The nephron, (D), is the functional unit of the kidney. Glucagon, (C), is a pancreatic hormone.

18. **(B) Density** The question asks what property is affected when mass is held constant but volume is changed. Recall that density is defined as mass over volume, so if mass is held constant and volume is changed, the density will also change. It gets larger when the volume is decreased and smaller when the volume is increased.

19. **(A) Active immunity** This question is asking about the body's response to a live pathogen. Recall that pathogens trigger the immune system to create antibodies as well as memory B-cells and T-cells. These memory cells will respond to that specific pathogen if it is detected again in the future, there by establishing active immunity, choice **(A)**. Passive immunity, (B), is produced from exposure to antibodies, not the pathogen. By definition, an antigen, (C), is any substance that triggers an immune response. Autoimmune diseases, (D), occur when an immune response is triggered against the body's own cells.

20. **(A) Herniated lumbar disc** This question tests your ability to infer a logical cause-and-effect relationship. The term "sciatica" refers to the sciatic nerve, which is the largest single nerve in the human body and branches from the lower spine into the buttocks and legs. If you did not recall the anatomy of the sciatic nerve, because the symptom is pain "that shoots from the lower back through the hips and legs," you could infer the problem likely relates to a spinal nerve. The most likely cause of the symptoms would be a problem in the upper lumbar or lower thoracic discs, so choice **(A)** is correct. The coccyx (tailbone) is at the lowest end of the spine and is not the site of any spinal nerves, so damage there is not likely to cause the noted symptoms; eliminate (B). A bruised calf muscle would cause pain in the lower leg only, so (C) is incorrect. A myocardial infarction (commonly called a "heart attack," as the root *cardia* suggests) would not produce pain in the lower body, so eliminate (D).

21. **(D) There is no correlation between the candidate's popularity and voters' education.** The campaign manager wants to find out whether the candidate is equally popular among voters at all educational levels or whether she is more popular among voters with less education. The question asks for an appropriate null hypothesis for the manager's study. A null hypothesis states that there is no relationship between variables. In this case, the variables under study are the candidate's popularity and voter education level. Choice **(D)** correctly states that there is no relationship between these two variables. Choice (A) states a possible research, or experimental, hypothesis—that there is a relationship between the variables. Choice (B) makes a statement about other candidates, which is not the topic of the proposed poll. While there may be a direct relationship between voter income and education, the poll will examine the relationship between education and attitude toward this candidate, so choice (C) is incorrect.

22. **(C) Sarcomere** This question is asking about the anatomy of smooth muscle. Recall that smooth muscle is unstriated muscle that does not have individual neuromuscular junctions. Actin and myosin, choices (A) and (B) respectively, are

present in smooth muscle tissue, but they are *not* arranged into sarcomeres; this is why smooth muscle does not appear striated. The same logic confirms choice **(C)** as correct. Gap junctions, (D), occur in both smooth and cardiac muscle tissue, where they allow cells to contract in tandem.

23. **(C) It would melt to form the denser liquid state.** This question requires usage of the figure provided. According to the phase diagram, water is liquid at high pressures since the solid liquid line has a negative slope. Thus, if pressure were increased but temperature remained the same, solid ice would melt to liquid water since the liquid form is denser. Solids are not compressible, so the water will not change volume to become more dense—eliminate (A). Choice (B) is opposite to the correct answer because the liquid state is more dense.

24. **(C) Salt decreases the freezing point of water, enabling it to melt at lower temperatures.** Based on the information in the table, as more salt is added, the freezing point of water decreases. A lower freezing point means that the ice will melt at a lower temperature. Choices (A) and (D) can be eliminated since the addition of salt decreases, not increases, the freezing point. Choice (B) can also be eliminated since a decrease in freezing point would cause ice to melt at lower, not higher, temperatures.

25. **(D) Deposition** This question is asking for the process that does not require an input of heat. Recall that heat must be added to go from a solid to a liquid to a gas. Deposition, going from gas straight to a solid, will release heat. Melting, (A), going from solid to liquid; sublimation, (B), going from solid to gas; and vaporization, (C), going from liquid to gas, all require heat input.

26. **(D) Preventing the activation of cytotoxic T-cells** This question is asking about the final stage of HIV infection, otherwise known as acquired immune deficiency syndrome (AIDS). Recall that the HIV virus replicates inside, and thus destroys, helper T-cells, so you can predict the answer will relate to the role of these cells. This matches choice **(D)**. Helper T-cells produce cytokines that activate the cytotoxic T-cells. Choice (C) describes the cause of allergies, and (B) describes the changes that occur as antigen levels subside in a functioning immune system. The adaptive immune system responds to antigen signatures, as in choice (A).

27. **(B) Protects the body against dehydration** This question is asking about the role of the integumentary system. Recall that the integumentary system consists of the skin, hair, nails, and sweat glands. Predict that the integumentary system acts as a barrier against the outside world. Choice **(B)** matches this prediction, as the skin is a waterproof barrier that prevents

excessive fluid loss. While some fluid is lost through the sweat glands, it is the genitourinary system (choices (A) and (D)) that controls blood volume by regulating fluid loss. Choice (C) describes a role of the endocrine system.

28. **(C) Call prices are positively, linearly related to stock prices and positively, but not linearly, related to days remaining.** Note that you do not need to know anything about investing in the stock market to answer this question. Focus on what is being tested, which is the relationship between a dependent variable and two independent variables. Everything needed to determine the correct answer is contained within the question and table.

The question states that call prices are a dependent variable and the price of the underlying stock and the days remaining until expiration are independent variables. The accompanying chart displays some values of these three variables. The question asks you to determine which of the answer choices correctly describes the relationships among the variables. To determine the relationship of a dependent variable to a particular independent variable when there are multiple independent variables, hold the other independent variables constant. There are three table rows with 30 days remaining. The stock prices for those entries are $20, $40, and $60 and the call prices are $1, $2, and $3. So, if the days remaining are held constant at 30, the option price is $\frac{1}{20}$ of the stock price, and the relationship between these two variable is positive and linear. Eliminate choices (A) and (D). Similarly, for a stock price of $20, as the days remaining go from 30 to 60 to 90, the call prices are $1.00, $1.75, and $2.00. When the stock price increases from $30 to $60, the call price increases $0.75, but when the stock goes up another $30 to $90, the call price increases $1.25. Therefore, call prices are positively, but not linearly, related to days remaining, and choice **(C)** is correct.

29. **(A) Superior and ventral** This question is asking where the sternum is located in relation to the coronal and transverse planes. Recall that the sternum is located in the top half of the body in the front, so it is on the superior side of the transverse plane and on the ventral side of the coronal plane.

30. **(B) Urea** This question is asking about the normal components of urine. Recall that the body excretes wastes that have been filtered from the blood through the urine, so predict that the answer is a waste product. This matches choice **(B)**. Urea is a metabolic byproduct that is removed from the blood by the kidneys. Glucose, (A), in the urine can be an indication of diabetes. The presence of blood cells, (C), or protein (amino acids), (D), in the urine could indicate kidney damage.

31. (C) The semilunar valves open under increased pressure. This question is asking about ventricular systole. Recall that systole indicates a contraction of the heart muscle, so predict that the answer will refer to what occurs as the ventricles contract. This matches answer choice **(C)**: as the ventricles contract, the increased pressure forces open the semilunar valves, allowing blood to be ejected from the heart into the arteries. Atrial systole forces open the AV valves, as in choice (D), and ejects blood into the ventricle, (B). The ventricle is relaxed, (A), during ventricular diastole.

32. (A) He equated correlation with causation. The question describes a study that found a group of people who experience chronic pain were less happy than a comparable group that were not experiencing chronic pain. The researcher concluded that unhappiness "is a major cause of chronic pain." The question asks for the flaw in the researcher's reasoning. Although the numerical results do suggest a positive correlation between chronic pain and unhappiness, nothing in the study indicates whether sadness caused pain, pain caused sadness, or some third variable caused both. Choice **(A)** is correct. The fact that the two groups in the study had "the same demographic characteristics" discredits choice (B). If a study is properly performed, one study can test (but not prove) a hypothesis, so eliminate (C). Choice (D) is intriguing because no mention is made of the researcher's initial hypothesis, null or otherwise. Nevertheless, the presence or absence of the null hypothesis was not the reason for the researcher's unsupported conclusion.

33. (D) Sympathetic and parasympathetic This question is asking about homeostatic regulation. Recall that *homeostasis* refers to maintaining a stable internal environment. Predict that homeostasis is regulated by the two divisions of the autonomic nervous system that work in opposition to one another: sympathetic and parasympathetic. This matches answer choice **(D)**. The sympathetic division causes "fight or flight" responses, and the parasympathetic returns the body to its resting state.

34. (A) Salivating This question is asking for an activity that is part of chemical digestion. Recall that chemical digestion is the process by which food is broken down at the molecular level by acids, bases, or enzymes, so predict that the answer will involve a chemical agent. Choice **(A)** matches this prediction. Saliva contains two enzymes that break down carbohydrates and lipids. Choices (B) and (C), swallowing and chewing respectively, are examples of mechanical digestion. Belching could occur when stomach gasses build up as the result of digestion, but it is not a digestive process.

35. (B) Gastric acid The question asks you to identify which of the answer choices is *not* made up of macromolecules. Recall that the four most common macromolecules in biology are carbohydrates, lipids, proteins, and nucleic acids, so the correct answer will be a substance that is not one of these. Gastric acid is composed of three simple compounds, HCl, KCl, and NaCl, none of which are macromolecules, so choice **(B)** is correct. The other choices are all macromolecular substances.

36. (A) A decrease in blood glucose stimulates glucagon; an increase in blood glucose stimulates insulin. This question is asking about the regulation of blood glucose levels. Recall that blood glucose is regulated by two opposing hormones—glucose and insulin—operating as a negative feedback loop, and that insulin stimulates the cells to uptake glucose. Glucagon acts in an antagonistic fashion, meaning it acts to oppose insulin. Choice **(A)** matches this prediction. Glucagon is secreted when blood glucose is low; it causes glucose to be released from the cells, raising blood sugar levels. When blood sugar levels are high, insulin is secreted to lower the levels. Choice (B) is partly true; an increase in insulin lowers blood glucose. However, it is a *decrease* in blood glucose that stimulates glucagon. Choices (C) and (D) describe the opposite of what occurs.

37. (B) 3, 2, 6 The question shows a chemical equation with the numbers of both reactants and one product missing. Your task is to find the coefficients that are needed to balance the equation. Since the coefficient of $Hg_3(PO_4)_2$ is known to be 1 because there is no blank preceding it, that is a good place to start. In order to get 3 atoms of Hg as a product of the reaction, there must be the same number in the reactants. The only source of this component is $Hg(OH)_2$, so the first missing number is 3. Similarly, 2 atoms of P are required because the subscript 2 applies to everything inside the parentheses, so the second blank is 2. Next look at H. There are $3 \times 2 = 6$ H in the first reactant and another 6 in the second reactant for a total of 12 H. Thus, 6 H_2O will balance the equation, and choice **(B)** is correct. Verify this answer by checking the number of O. There are $3 \times 2 = 6$ plus $2 \times 4 = 8$ for a total of 14 O on the input side, and $4 \times 2 = 8$ plus $6 \times 1 = 6$ for a total of 14 on the output side—the O balances.

38. (B) Tarsal This question is asking you to correctly identify a short bone. Recall that short bones are wider than they are long. The tarsals of the foot are short bones. The phalanges of the fingers and toes, choice (A), are long bones; the scapula of the shoulder, (C), is a flat bone; and the radius of the forearm, (D), is a long bone.

39. (A) Luteinizing hormone This question is asking you to identify the hormone that induces ovulation. Recall that a spike in luteinizing hormone at day 14 in the menstrual cycle will trigger ovulation. Estrogen, choice (B), triggers the thickening of the endometrium, and progesterone, (D), maintains it. The corpus luteum, (C), is not a hormone. Instead, it is the remaining tissue after the follicle ruptures.

40. (D) Increasing the concentration of oxygen in the blood Recall that the rate of diffusion is proportional to the concentration gradient and to the surface area. To decrease the rate, either the concentration gradient or surface area must be smaller. The air always contains more oxygen than the blood, but by increasing the concentration of oxygen in the blood, the difference in concentration between the air and the blood becomes smaller, thus decreasing the rate of diffusion.

41. (C) Milliliters The question mentions a dosage amount in deciliters and asks what unit should be used to ensure that the dosage is accurate to within $\pm 1\%$ when measured to the nearest whole number. A deciliter is 0.1 L, and 1% converts to 0.01, so the required degree of accuracy is 0.1 L $\times$ 0.01 = 0.001 L, which is one-thousandth of a liter. The prefix for thousandth is *milli*, so choice **(C)** is correct.

42. (D) Liver This question is asking about bile production. Recall and predict that bile is produced in the liver, choice **(D)**. Bile is stored in the gall bladder, (A). It passes through the bile duct, (B), and is secreted into the duodenum (C).

43. (A) Fallopian tubes, site of fertilization This question is asking which reproductive structure is correctly paired with its function. Recall that follicles mature in the ovaries and fertilization of the ovum occurs in the fallopian tubes. Sperm are produced in the testes, and the prostate and seminal vesicles produce the nourishing and lubricating fluids for the sperm.

44. (C) The black-furred parent has a recessive white fur allele. The question states that white fur is a recessive trait and that a black-furred parent and a white-furred parent have a white-furred offspring. You must select the answer that is a valid deduction. Because white fur is a recessive trait, any white-furred member of the species must have two white fur alleles; this applies to both the white-furred parent and the offspring. Thus, the offspring must have acquired a white fur allele from the black parent. The black-furred parent must, therefore, have the recessive white fur gene, making choice **(C)** correct. The traits of one offspring have no bearing on the traits of subsequent offspring, so eliminate choice (A). The question states that the white fur allele is the recessive one, so (B) is incorrect. As already predicted, a white-furred animal of this species must have two white fur alleles; (D) is incorrect.

45. (D) Veins This question is asking about the anatomical presence of valves in blood vessels. Recall that valves prevent the backflow of blood. Because the blood pressure is lower as blood is returned to the heart, you could predict that valves will be present in the blood vessels of the venous system. Choice **(D)** matches your prediction.

46. (B) $R = \dfrac{r_1 r_2}{r_1 + r_2}$ A class conducts an experiment to determine how placing different resistors in parallel affects the total resistance of a circuit. Voltage (V), which is held constant, is set by the researchers. The researchers also choose the resistors, r_1 and r_2. As the students place different resistors in parallel, they measure current flow (I). Then Ohm's law, $V = IR$, allows total resistance, R, to be calculated. The question asks for an equation that represents a hypothesis the class could be testing. Recall that a hypothesis is about the effects of independent variables on a dependent variable.

Choice (A) restates Ohm's law, which is a given, so it is not the hypothesis. Choice (C) merely rearranges Ohm's law. Eliminate these choices. Choice (D) calculates r_1 in terms of the other resistor and total resistance. But r_1 is known and controlled by the experimenters; after all, they choose each resistor to place in the circuit. This is not a dependent variable in this experiment. Choice **(B)** predicts that the resistance calculated using Ohm's law will be the product of the two resistors divided by their sum, and this is a hypothesis about the response of a dependent variable to manipulation of independent variables that can be tested by this experiment.

47. (D) The diaphragm and intercostal muscles relax, decreasing pressure in the lungs. The question pertains to muscle contraction and air pressure in the lungs. During inhalation, the diaphragm and intercostal muscles simultaneously relax, increasing the volume of the lungs, causing the pressure to drop. Air will subsequently flow into the lungs.

48. (C) There is no apparent correlation between temperature and the number of bluebirds observed. The scatterplot shows the data gathered by a bird-watcher, and you must identify the relationship between those two variables. Examine the pattern of the data points. There were three days when six or more birds were seen, and the temperatures on those days varied widely. Similarly, the recorded temperatures ranged from just over 40°F to 70°F on the days when only one bird was spotted. Thus, there is no discernible relationship between bluebirds and temperature; choice **(C)** is correct.

49. (C) Plasma cells This question is asking about the immune response to a new pathogen. Recall that a new pathogen would trigger the innate immune system. Therefore, predict that the answer will be a component of the adaptive immune system or not be a part of the immune system at all. Choice **(C)** is a match. Plasma cells are differentiated B-cells that produce antibodies after being exposed to a known antigen. Macrophages, (A); NK lympocytes, (B); and dendritic cells, (D), are all leukocytes of the innate immune system.

50. **(C) Liver** Because this question is asking about which organ does *not* secrete a hormone involved in nutrient absorption/distribution, you can predict that three of the answer choices will secrete hormones involved in digestion. Gastrin, a hormone that stimulates the release of HCl, is secreted by the stomach and the duodenum (part of the small intestine), as in choices (A) and (D), respectively. Secretin, a hormone that stimulates the release of pancreatic enzymes, is secreted from the pancreas, (B), as well as from the duodenum, (D). Other hormones with roles in digestion include insulin and glucagon (both from the pancreas) and cholecystokinin (CCK, from the small intestine). The liver, choice **(C)**, creates bile, a key digestive enzyme but *not* a digestive hormone.

51. **(D) T-cells** This question is asking about one part of the immune system. Recall that the adaptive immune system responds to specific antigens. This is in contrast to the innate immune system, which has a nonspecific response. T-cells are activated by the presence of specific antigens, so choice **(D)** is correct. Phagocytes, (A), ingest a variety of detritus in the blood, including dead cells and pathogens. Inflammation and earwax, choices (C) and (D) respectively, are part of the innate immune system.

52. **(B) Increase in blood pH** This question is asking what happens during hyperventilation that would lead to a decrease in respiration rate. The medulla oblongata in the brain stem changes respiration rate in response to changes in blood pH. Hyperventilation would lead to a large drop in blood CO_2 levels, causing the concentration of H^+ and HCO_3^- to drop, resulting in an increase in blood pH. In response, the medulla oblongata would decrease the respiration rate.

53. **(A) Osteoclasts** The question asks what type of cells break down bone. Recall that osteoclasts break down or cleave bone. Osteoblasts, choice (C), help to build bone, and an osteocyte, (B), is the most common cell in mature bone. Osteons, (D), are not cells but are cylindrical structures within compact bone.

English and Language Usage

1. **(B) :** This sentence begins with an independent clause (if a period followed "supplies," the sentence would express a complete thought. However, the missing punctuation mark introduces a list of items that could not stand alone as another sentence. The colon in choice **(B)** is the correct punctuation mark to introduce a list after an independent clause.

2. **(D) ballpark figure** The question indicates that the sentence has informal usage in it, so read looking for figures of speech that would not be appropriate for formal academic writing. The phrase "ballpark figure" in choice **(D)** is an informal expression that means "rough estimate." The other phrases in the answer choices are examples of formal or standard uses of the English language.

3. **(A) are** The subject of the sentence is the plural noun "producers." The missing word is part of the verb, which must agree in number with the subject. Choice (B) is incorrect because it is singular. Choice (C), "will," might be tempting because the new film will be released in the future. However, "will planning" is not the correct form of the future tense for an ongoing action; "will be planning" would be needed. Choice **(A)** correctly uses the plural "are," and it places the planning for the future release of the film in the present, a logical order of events.

4. **(D) Change "there" to "their."** In this sentence, the correct homophone is the plural possessive pronoun *their*.

5. **(C) Scientific report** Different publications require different writing styles for the intended audience to understand and appreciate the information. The tone, subject matter, and word choice of a piece of writing can indicate the type of publication in which it did or should appear. The sentence in this question, about a scientific study, is written in a formal tone using scientific wording such as "subjects" (instead of *people*). This type of text would most likely appear in a scientific report, choice **(C)**.

6. **(B) Because** The missing word introduces a subordinate or dependent clause and must express the cause-and-effect relationship between the act of leaving the water on and the overflowing of the sink. Only choice **(B)** properly expresses the relationship between the dependent clause and the independent clause.

7. **(D) Denied** The prefix *dis-* suggests reversal or removal, which indicates the meaning will be close to the opposite of *claim*. To "unclaim" knowledge is to *deny* knowledge, and choice **(D)**, "Denied," is a match. If the researcher had "proclaimed" his knowledge of wrongdoing, he would have announced it.

8. **(A) Walter stepped out of the office building and walked toward his car, careful not to slip on the thin layer of ice that covered the parking lot.** A novel is a written narrative that tells the story of fictional characters and events. The style is typically descriptive, and the tone can vary depending on the subject matter. Choice **(A)** is the sentence most likely to be found in a novel because it narrates the actions of a specific character

and has a descriptive style. Choice (B) refers to recent events related to a crime and would likely be found in a news report. The tone of choice (C) is very formal and contains jargon that would likely be found in a business memo. Choice (D) is also formal, but the factual content indicates that it belongs in a scientific article.

9. **(A) Free** The prefixes *dis-* and *en-* are attached to the root word *tangle*. *En* + *tangle* means "tangled together." *Dis* + *en* + *tangle* means the opposite: "not tangled together." Choice **(A)**, "Free," matches this prediction. Context clues are helpful as well: the words "caught" and "snare" indicate being trapped, so you can infer that Marcus is attempting to "free" the fawn.

10. **(A) its ; her** A glance at the answer choices indicates that this question deals with pronoun rules. The first blank requires a singular, neuter pronoun to refer to its antecedent, "team." The second blank needs a singular, female, possessive pronoun because it is referring to each individual player on the girls' team.

11. **(C) Although free parking might draw more patrons to the downtown stores, the city cannot afford to lose any parking revenue.** A complex sentence is composed of an independent clause and a least one dependent clause. Choices (A) and (D) are simple sentences because they each only contain one independent clause. Choice (B) is comprised of two independent clauses joined by "and," so it is a compound sentence. In choice **(C)**, the first clause is dependent, since it does not express a complete thought by itself, while the second clause could stand alone as a complete sentence, making it independent.

12. **(C) Everyone who lost points on the test have to stay after class.** Analyze each sentence for subject-verb agreement; a singular subject requires a singular verb, and a plural subject requires a plural verb. You are looking for the *incorrect* example. In choice (A), the past tense verb "went" can be paired with either a singular or a plural subject, so this sentence is correct as written. The subject of the sentence in choice (B) is "boy," which correctly agrees with the singular verb "is going." In choice (D), the plural subject "cheerleaders" agrees with the plural verb "are leading." The subject of the sentence in choice **(C)** is the singular pronoun "everyone," which does not agree in number with the plural verb "have."

13. **(C) Types of research include quantitative and qualitative methods.** The title of this sample outline indicates that it presents ways to conduct research. The items are listed in a logical fashion, using heading levels to indicate relationships. The outline indicates that both quantitative and qualitative meth-

ods are available to researchers, not that they need to choose one or the other, as in choice (A). Application and description are separate categories, so eliminate (B). Quantitative methods are listed first, but this does not imply that they are preferable to qualitative methods; eliminate (D).

14. **(C) Complyant** Each of these words involves a spelling rule that frequently causes trouble. The root word of choice (B), *enjoy*, correctly follows the rule for adding a suffix to a word that ends in *-oy*. Choices (A), (C), and (D) have root words that end in *y* preceded by a consonant (*rely, comply, deny*). Only **(C)** fails to follow the rule for adding a suffix beginning with a vowel, which is to change the *y* to *i*.

15. **(B) After Jarvis dropped the expensive laptop, everyone in the cafeteria turned around and stared at him.** The correct answer needs to convey the same meaning as the original sentences. Choice **(B)** conveys the information clearly and fluently, in the correct sequence. Choice (A) uses passive voice and lacks a comma after "Jarvis," which is needed because this answer choice is a compound sentence. Choice (C) also uses passive voice, and by placing the ideas in short modifying clauses, it produces a choppy effect. Choice (D) changes the meaning by using "because" to introduce a cause-and-effect relationship between the cost of the laptop and people turning to look; they may well have turned around because they heard the loud noise of some object falling without knowing what it was, let alone whether it was expensive.

16. **(D) weary.** If you are not certain of the meaning of "lethargic," use context clues to predict the correct answer. The phrase "took a nap" suggests that Ria was tired, so you can infer that feeling "lethargic" means being "tired." Choice **(D)**, "weary," is a match. If you read the word "weary" back into the sentence in place of "lethargic," it makes sense.

17. **(C) uncertain.** The context clues suggest that a precarious situation is one in which it is difficult to know how to behave or proceed. "Uncertain" is a match for this prediction.

18. **(B) The comma after "freedom"** This question asks about punctuation, and the sentence contains a number of commas and one semicolon. The semicolon is used correctly to join two independent clauses that express closely related thoughts. The comma in choice **(B)** incorrectly separates the two terms of the compound direct object—"freedom" and "discipline."

19. **(D) had drunk** This question is testing two important concepts—verb tense and irregular verb forms. To determine the tense of the missing verb, analyze the context clues and decide the logical order of the events described in the sentence. In this sentence, Dana did something with water prior

to running. When an action is completed prior to another past action, past perfect tense is correct. Eliminate choices (A) and (C). The verb *to drink* is an irregular verb that changes its spelling to "drank" in past tense and "drunk" in the past perfect tense. Choice **(D)** uses the proper tense and correct spelling of the verb *to drink* for this sentence.

20. **(C) veins** The context clues suggest the correct word relates to a blood vessel; of the homophones *vanes*, *vain*, and *vein*, only choice **(C)** is a type of blood vessel. With an apostrophe, the word "vein's" is singular and possessive; a correct construction with this word would be "The vein's lining may become irritated."

21. **(C) Finally, if the expanded trial succeeds, the FDA should consider approving the new drug.** This question tests your understanding of paragraph structure. The paragraph gives details of a drug trial that has taken place and of a proposed trial of the drug. The concluding sentence will provide a logical next step in the sequence of events or outcome of the series of trials. Choice **(C)** begins with the key word "finally," indicating that it is a concluding statement, and this sentence recommends a future action based on what has come before. The other choices offer supporting details about the clinical study and the drug.

22. **(A) their ; they're** The answer choices in this sentence are all homophones, meaning they sound alike but have different spellings, definitions, and even parts of speech. The context clues in the sentence help clarify which word is needed in each blank. The first blank requires a possessive adjective, narrowing the choices down to (A) and (B). The second blank must include a subject and helping verb, so the contraction *they're*, short for "they are," in choice **(A)** is correct.

23. **(B) Knowledge of an event before it happens** The root and affixes suggest "prescience" most nearly means "knowing" (*sci*), "before" (*pre-*), and "the state of something" (*-ence*). Thus, predict this word means "knowing something beforehand." This matches choice **(B)** very well.

24. **(D) scratching her head** This question asks about informal usage, so read the sentence looking for language that would not be appropriate for formal academic writing. The phrase

"scratching her head" is an informal, figurative expression that is used to describe confusion in response to a unexpected situation.

25. **(D) uncertainty.** "Trusted" provides a context clue; because he trusts her, Gregory is likely to be certain or confident in Kiera's sincerity. Therefore, the phrase "without reservation" most likely means "without condition" or "with certainty." To act "with certainty" means to act "without uncertainty," making choice **(D)** the correct answer. A reservation can be a thing that is set aside, or assigned, for some use (e.g., "We have a table reserved for dinner"), but that meaning does not fit the context here, making (A) incorrect.

26. **(A) When she found her brother outside, Julie exclaimed, "Michael, there you are! A short while ago, mother said, 'Children, come inside.'"** Recall that in direct dialogue, the quoted text is separated from the speaker by a comma. The sentence in choice **(A)** correctly introduces Julie's quote and the quote inside her quote with a comma. The quotation of the mother's words is properly offset with a pair of single quotation marks.

27. **(A) Similarly** The blank in the sentence must be filled by a transition word that links a sentence about one study to a sentence about another study. Both studies support the idea that lack of sleep affects people's cognitive skills. The word "Similarly" reflects this relationship between the sentences. All the other answer choices would signal contrasting ideas.

28. **(C) The rusty old boat with the torn sails** The complete subject of a sentence includes the simple subject and all words and phrases in the sentence that describe it. In this sentence, "boat" is the simple subject. The article "The," the adjectives "rusty" and "old," and the prepositional phrase "with the torn sails" all serve to describe the boat.

Kaplan Study Planner for the TEAS

For each test content area—*Reading*, *Mathematics*, *Science*, and *English language and usage*—write the number of questions you answered correctly in the second column. For purposes of this diagnostic test, count all of the questions toward your score.

To calculate the percentage correct for each content area, enter the number of questions you got right in the numerator (top part) of the fraction. Then do the calculations: divide the number you got right by the number of questions in the content area and multiply that result by 100. Follow the same procedure for calculating your overall percentage; here you are dividing by the number of questions on the entire test, which is 170.

Content Area	# Correct	% Correct
Reading	___ out of 53	$100 \times \dfrac{}{53} = $ ___ %
Mathematics	___ out of 36	$100 \times \dfrac{}{36} = $ ___ %
Science	___ out of 53	$100 \times \dfrac{}{53} = $ ___ %
English and language usage	___ out of 28	$100 \times \dfrac{}{28} = $ ___ %
Total	___ out of 170	$100 \times \dfrac{}{170} = $ ___ %

Then with your studying, target the content areas where you have the most opportunity to improve your score. Note that if a school to which you are applying considers scores in each content area, then you will want to focus most on the content areas in which you missed the greatest *percentage* of correct answers. However, if a school considers the composite (overall) score, then focusing on the areas in which you missed the greatest *number* of questions can raise your composite score the most.

Reading

Understanding written material will be critical to your success in a nursing or health science program and to your ability to care for clients as a health care professional. Whether reading a textbook, a patient's chart, a healthcare facility's policies, or research study results, you will need to be able to grasp an author's main idea and purpose in writing, evaluate trends or patterns in words and data, focus on important details, draw appropriate conclusions on the basis of what you've read, and apply information and conclusions to your work. The TEAS *Reading* content area tests your ability to perform these tasks.

Questions by Content Area

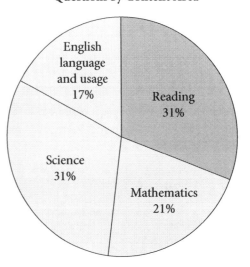

The TEAS Reading Content Area

Of the 170 items on the TEAS, 53 will be in the *Reading* content area, and you will have 64 minutes to answer them.

While you have on average just over a minute per question, most questions will require reading a short passage or a figure or table first. As a rule of thumb, if you invest about 45 seconds in reading a paragraph of text, a table, or a figure and take about 30 seconds to answer each question, you will stay on pace to complete the *Reading* section.

> *Example:* A three-paragraph text passage has four questions associated with it.
>
> 45 seconds × 3 paragraphs = 2 minutes 15 seconds
>
> 30 seconds × 4 questions = 2 minutes
>
> Reading the passage and answering four questions takes 4 minutes 15 seconds.

Of course, some passages, tables, and figures are very short and will take much less than 45 seconds to read, while others are longer and will require more time to map. Some questions will not refer to any information beyond what's in the question itself. The key is to work at a steady pace. Reading in a hurry because you are worried about time will lead to choosing wrong answers.

Of the 53 *Reading* questions, 47 will be scored and 6 will be unscored. You won't know which questions are unscored, so do your best on every question.

The 47 scored *Reading* questions come from three sub-content areas:

Sub-content Areas	# of Questions
Key ideas and details	22
Craft and structure	14
Integration of knowledge and ideas	11

Kaplan's *High-Yield Practice for the New ATI TEAS®* includes a chapter covering the area of *Reading* the TEAS tests most:

- Chapter 1: Main Ideas and Supporting Details

The Kaplan Method for Reading

Reading on the TEAS requires a **strategic** approach. Following the Kaplan Method for Reading helps you get the correct answer efficiently, without wasting time.

KAPLAN METHOD FOR READING

Step 1: Read the stimulus strategically.*

Step 2: Analyze the question.

Step 3: Research.

Step 4: Predict the answer.

Step 5: Evaluate the answer choices.

* If there is only one question on a stimulus, switch the order of steps 1 and 2. If there is no stimulus, begin with Step 2.

Step 1: Read the stimulus strategically.

The *stimulus* is the passage, figure, or chart on which the questions are based. Reading *strategically* means paying special attention to the **topic** and **scope** of the stimulus. The topic is the subject the author is writing about, and the scope is the specific aspect of that topic in which the author is interested. In a passage, the topic and scope are often found in the first few sentences. In a figure or graph, they are often found in the title, headings, and labels. Also, seek to understand the author's **purpose** in writing. Often, this is to explain a process, describe a topic, or outline information, but sometimes the author is presenting a particular point of view or seeking to persuade the reader.

When the stimulus is a passage of more than a few sentences or a figure or table of any complexity, you should also take notes as you read. Your notes should sum up the important ideas of the stimulus. Write notes in your own words and use abbreviations and symbols. Your notes become a **map** of the stimulus, both summarizing important information and helping you find details to answer questions. Investing time in understanding the stimulus helps you answer the questions more efficiently.

Note: Some questions do not refer to a stimulus. When this is the case, proceed directly to step 2. Also, if there is only one question on a stimulus, read the question first (step 2) and then read the stimulus strategically as you research the answer to that question (combining steps 1 and 3).

Step 2: Analyze the question.

Determine exactly what the question asks you to find. Is it asking for the author's main point or primary purpose in writing? Or is it asking for a detail from the stimulus? Or is it asking you to make an inference based on the stimulus? Or is it asking why the author included some detail or feature? How you research your map and the stimulus and what you will look for in a correct answer depend on the task in the question.

Step 3: Research.

Research the answer in the stimulus. If you mapped it in step 1, your map will help you find the right place quickly; read your notes and, as needed, the appropriate portion of the stimulus.

If you are reading the stimulus for the first time, because there is only one question on the stimulus, then make sure to read it strategically. Many TEAS questions require you to grasp the big picture of a stimulus, interpret a detail in context, or connect the dots between different details.

Step 4: Predict the answer.

Before looking at the answer choices, *predict* the correct answer. Having the answer clearly in mind before looking at the choices will help you choose the correct answer and not be misled by choices that "sound right" but aren't actually correct.

Some questions are open-ended and don't allow for a precise prediction. Examples are "Based on the passage, what conclusion can you reasonably draw?" or "Which of the following questions are answered by the passage?" Even in these cases, you can review your map and prepare a mental checklist of the important ideas and information in the stimulus. The correct answer will align with one of those.

Step 5: Evaluate the answer choices.

Evaluate the answer choices looking for a match for your prediction and eliminating choices that do not match. If the answer you expected is not there, revisit Steps 2–4 to refine your thinking.

MAIN IDEAS AND SUPPORTING DETAILS

LEARNING OBJECTIVES

- Identify the author's main idea and the details used to support that idea
- Identify the relevant information to answer a question
- Make logical inferences based on information provided
- Use the relationship of events in a sequence to answer a question or achieve a result

Of the 47 scored *Reading* questions, 22 (47%) will be in the sub-content area of *Key ideas and details*. With these questions, the TEAS tests your ability to read for the "big picture" and for important details, as well as to draw inferences from your reading and apply what you learn from text.

This chapter addresses these skills in four lessons:

Lesson 1: Strategic Reading

Lesson 2: Reading for Details

Lesson 3: Making Inferences

Lesson 4: Understanding Sequences of Events

Questions by Sub-content Area

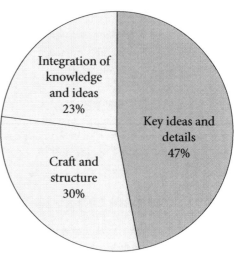

LESSON 1

Strategic Reading

LEARNING OBJECTIVES

- Identify the author's main idea
- Identify supporting details

Main Idea

Many TEAS questions ask you to identify the main idea, which is the subject the author is writing about or the point he or she is making in the stimulus. You can identify the main idea by asking yourself, "What does the author want me to know?" You should also ask, "Why does the author want me to know it?" Sometimes the writer will be simply describing or explaining a topic, and other times the author will be trying to persuade you of a particular point of view.

The correct answer to a question about the main idea, topic, or author's primary purpose in writing is broad enough to reflect the entire stimulus, but not so broad that it goes beyond the author's point. Eliminate answer choices that are supporting details; these answers are too narrow.

Supporting Details

Other questions ask about details the author includes to support the main idea. Details are explicitly stated in the stimulus, and important details in passages—the kind of details you are likely to see a question about—are usually indicated by keywords indicating contrast, emphasis, or a sequence. Contrast keywords, which signal a different idea or example, include "however" or "on the other hand." "Especially" or "surprisingly" are examples of emphasis key words, signaling a fact or idea the author thinks is important. Words like "first," "second," and "third" or a series of dates indicate a sequence of events or steps. Details may also be highlighted by structural features of the text, like headings.

Follow along as a TEAS expert answers first a main idea question and then a supporting detail question.

> Like most superheroes, the Incredible Hulk possesses supernatural abilities. Among other talents, he has unlimited strength and the ability to leap several miles. Though theoretically capable of great evil, he is on the side of good, an especially important position given the time in which he first appeared in Marvel comics. First created at the height of post–World War II paranoia about nuclear war, the Incredible Hulk stories offer a fascinating look at the dual nature of human beings. On the one hand, he is a mild-mannered, bespectacled scientist. On the other, he is a raging, rampaging beast. More than a statement about the dangers of the Atomic Age, the Hulk is a reflection of the two sides in each of us—the calm, logical human and the raging animal.

Question	Analysis
	Step 1: The author begins by describing the Incredible Hulk. This description lays the foundation for the author to argue that the Incredible Hulk symbolizes the dual nature of human beings.
The author's primary purpose is	**Step 2**: This is a main idea question. Consider the entire passage to determine the author's purpose.
	Step 3: The author's main point is summarized in the last sentence. The other sentences in the paragraph are supporting details.
	Step 4: Predict that the correct answer is about what the Incredible Hulk symbolizes.
(A) to explain the confusion people can feel due to their dual nature.	**Step 5**: The author does not discuss any confusion people might feel about their dual nature.
(B) to argue that the Incredible Hulk symbolizes more than the particular concerns of his time.	Correct. This matches your prediction. The author's purpose is to argue that the Incredible Hulk symbolized not only post–World War II anxiety about nuclear war but also a more universal concern about human nature.
(C) to discuss the cultural and psychological importance of comic books in the post–World War II era.	The passage is not about comic books in general, only about the Incredible Hulk.
(D) to critique people's fears about nuclear war in the mid-twentieth century	This suggests that the author has an opinion about people's fears, but the author's opinion is about what the Incredible Hulk symbolized.

Here is a test expert's approach to a supporting detail question.

Question	Analysis
According to the author, the comic book character of the Incredible Hulk first appeared	**Step 2**: This question asks for a detail—information stated in the passage.
	Step 3: Your map shows that the relevant detail is in the middle of the paragraph, where the author places the superhero in historical context. The sentence with this detail begins: "First created at the height of post–World War II paranoia . . . ."

Question	Analysis
	Step 4: Predict an answer that restates this sentence.
(A) during a lull between wars.	**Step 5**: The passage does not mention a period between wars.
(B) after a nuclear attack.	The author notes anxiety about nuclear war but does not mention an actual nuclear attack.
(C) in a period of fear about nuclear war.	Correct. This choice matches your prediction.
(D) during a protest about atomic power.	The passage mentions fear of nuclear war but not protests over atomic power.

Now practice answering a main idea and a supporting detail question yourself. After reading and mapping the passage and answering each question, check your work against the explanations that follow.

In a remote valley of Baja California, Mexico, a small group of Kumeyaay Indians retain their traditional way of life. It was here that Eva Salazar learned the ancient art of basket weaving from her tribal elders. Among the Kumeyaay, women have the crucial responsibility of making baskets, which are important artifacts of everyday life. Kumeyaay baskets, tightly woven with expressive designs, were made mostly for utilitarian purposes—for cooking, storing food products in, gathering ingredients, and even, when turned upside down, wearing as hats. As traditional objects of art, they are also valued for their aesthetic beauty.

Following in her ancestors' footsteps, Eva Salazar uses traditional materials to weave her intricate baskets, primarily the strong, sharp reed known as juncus, as well as yucca, sumac, and other plants. She colors the reeds with black walnut, elderberry, and other natural dyes. Eva specializes in coiled baskets, made by starting the weaving at the bottom center of the basket and adding coils upward, then stitching the coils together. The shapes and decorations echo traditional forms. Her most ambitious work is a basket measuring almost three feet in diameter, which took her two years to weave and represents a masterpiece of Native American art.

Which of the following correctly states the main subject of the passage?

    (A)   Native American basket weaving
    (B)   A master basket weaver
    (C)   Uses of natural plants and dyes
    (D)   Kumeyaay traditions

Explanation

Step 1:

Topic: Kumeyaay Indian basket weaving
Scope: master weaver Eva Salazar
Purpose: inform
¶ 1: Importance and uses of baskets for the Kumeyaay
¶ 2: Eva Salazar—how she makes baskets

Step 2: This is a main idea question.

Step 3: Look at the topic and scope in your map to determine the main idea.

Step 4: Predict that the topic is Eva Salazar and her basket weaving.

Step 5: Only one answer choice mentions a specific basket weaver, so **(B)** is correct. Choice (A) is too broad. Choice (C) is a detail mentioned in the passage but not the main idea. Choice (D) goes beyond the point of the passage: the subject is basket weaving only, not all Kumeyaay traditions.

> The passage supports the statement that Salazar has followed in her ancestors' footsteps by stating that she
>
> (A)   mainly makes very large baskets.
> (B)   is also a skilled storyteller of traditional tales.
> (C)   uses natural materials and dyes.
> (D)   teaches basket weaving to college students.

Explanation

Step 1: The passage is the same as for the previous question.

Step 2: This question asks for a detail stated in the passage. The detail concerns Salazar's relationship with her ancestors.

Step 3: Your map shows you that details about Salazar are mostly in the second paragraph, so start your research there. The first two sentences are details about this master basket weaver "following in her ancestors' footsteps" by using traditional materials and dyes.

Step 4: Predict that the answer will have something to do with using traditional materials.

Step 5: The correct answer is choice **(C)**. None of the other answer choices matches your prediction.

KEY IDEAS

- Main idea questions ask about the overall topic or purpose of the passage.
- Supporting detail questions ask about evidence the author uses to develop the topic.
- Approach reading strategically, focusing on the passage's topic and scope and the author's purpose in writing.
- Make a prediction before evaluating the answer choices so you do not waste time thinking about or researching incorrect answers.

Strategic Reading Practice Questions

Questions 1–6 refer to the following passage.

In modern society, a form of folktale called the urban legend has emerged. These stories persist both for their entertainment value and for the transmission of popular values and beliefs. Urban legends are stories many have heard, claimed as true, but never actually verified. If you try to confirm one, it turns out that the people involved can never be found. Researchers of urban legends call the elusive participant in these supposedly "real-life" events a "FOAF": friend of a friend.

One classic urban legend involves alligators in the sewer systems of major metropolitan areas. According to the story, before alligators were a protected species, people vacationing in Florida purchased baby alligators to take home as souvenirs. After the novelty of having a pet alligator wore off, people would flush their souvenirs down the toilet. The baby alligators found a perfect growing environment in city sewer systems, where to this day they thrive on an ample supply of rats.

Urban legends also change with the times. In today's world of medical advances, one legend is that unsuspecting people are kidnapped, anesthetized, and subjected to an operation. They wake up with a kidney removed. Though even minimal research can dispel many legends, some seem plausible enough to be taken as true, at least initially. Occasionally, they have turned up on legitimate news broadcasts; more often, though, they are repeated through emails and social media.

1. The main focus of the passage is

   (A) traditional folktales.
   (B) urban legends.
   (C) friends of friends.
   (D) medical advances.

2. According to the passage, the successful urban legend contains all of the following characteristics EXCEPT

   (A) the topics of urban legends can change with the times.
   (B) messages that conform to popular values.
   (C) the qualities of a folktale.
   (D) a basis in reality.

3. Which of the following claims about urban legends is stated in the passage?

   (A) Their themes change with the times.
   (B) Most urban legends can be verified.
   (C) Urban legends are traditional forms of folklore.
   (D) Urban legends are mostly transmitted by national media.

4. The author of the passage is primarily concerned with

   (A) alligators living in Florida sewers.
   (B) kidney donors.
   (C) a new form of folklore.
   (D) researching urban legends.

5. According to the passage, urban legends are

   (A) restricted to cities.
   (B) easy to trace back to their source.
   (C) never taken seriously.
   (D) aligned with popular beliefs.

6. Which of the following is NOT explicitly stated in the passage?

   (A) Pet alligators were supposedly abandoned in sewers.
   (B) All urban legends instill fear in listeners.
   (C) Social media are frequent transmitters of urban legends.
   (D) Urban legends can be entertaining.

Review your work using the explanations in Part Six of this book.

LESSON 2

Reading for Details

LEARNING OBJECTIVES

- Identify the relevant information in text to answer a question
- Identify the relevant information in a graphic to answer a question

Details in Text

The TEAS tests your ability to glean relevant information from many different types of printed communication, including announcements, academic essays, advertisements, instructions, and memos. The test will include communications you might encounter in school, at work, or at home or around town.

Some TEAS questions require you to find specific information that is stated within a passage or depicted in a graphic. The TEAS will word these questions in a variety of ways:

> What reason does the author give to avoid mixing chemicals X and Y before sterilization?
>
> According to the passage, which of the following is a kind of ornament commonly found in Gothic cathedrals in England?
>
> At what time will the Annual General Meeting be held?

The correct answer to a detail question will be information or an idea that can be found in the stimulus. It may state the information using the same words as are in the stimulus, or it may paraphrase the information. Note that sometimes wrong answer choices will be information that is in the stimulus but do not answer the question asked. These choices might be tempting because they look familiar, but by analyzing the question to determine exactly what you are being asked for (step 2 of the Kaplan Method for Reading), you will avoid these traps.

Study how a TEAS expert would answer this detail question, one of several questions about the stimulus.

> To the Editor:
>
> Lately, there has been a good deal of discussion about whether or not a new bridge should be constructed over the Millville River. I firmly believe that this structure should be completed at the earliest opportunity, for some very good reasons. The current bridge is clearly decrepit, and indeed must be closed several months a year for much-needed maintenance. Our city should be embarrassed by the nuisance this inconvenience brings to commuters and tourists.
>
> Some might argue that our city cannot afford the considerable expense required for a bridge so far from the town center, but this concern can easily be dealt with. The state governor has made it clear that she considers infrastructure a matter of primary concern and will lobby the federal government for funding. And, as our city expands with new subdivisions providing housing to accommodate our booming population, the Millville River route will only see more and more traffic in the future.

Question	Analysis
	Step 1: Read the passage strategically. The letter has two paragraphs. The first states why the author believes a new bridge is needed. The second paragraph introduces a possible objection to the project—its expense—but dismisses this objection before moving on to a prediction about the city's population.
What does the letter writer say about the expense of constructing the new bridge?	**Step 2:** This is a detail question. You are looking for something the author says about the cost of the new bridge.
	Step 3: According to your passage map, information about cost is in paragraph 2—it's a possible barrier to construction. Research that paragraph.
	Step 4: The author states that the governor has prioritized the bridge project and will lobby for federal funds to pay for it. Look for an answer choice that says either the bridge will be expensive or that it will funded at least in part with federal dollars.
(A) It can be recouped by a newly instituted road tax.	A road tax is never mentioned in the letter. Eliminate.
(B) The high cost means the project will not proceed.	This prediction is contrary to the letter writer's opinion, which is that money can be found for the bridge.
(C) It can be met with federal funds.	Correct. This matches your prediction.
(D) It is the sole responsibility of the state.	Although the governor has said that infrastructure is a primary concern of the state, there is no suggestion that the state must be the sole funder. Indeed, the opposite is the case.

Now you try one. After answering the question, check your work against the explanation that follows.

First Annual Memorial Day Concert
Free to the Public!

When: May 26, noon to sunset

Where: Granville Park

Kickoff: Welcome speech from special guest Mayor Edugyan

Performances: The Campertown College Marching Band, the River Valley Elementary School Children's Choir, and Marco Whicker and the Sunset Singers

According to the poster, who will concert attendees see first on stage?

(A) The Campertown College Marching Band
(B) Marco Whicker and the Sunset Singers
(C) Mayor Edugyan
(D) This question cannot be answered from the information on the poster.

Explanation

Step 2: This is a detail question asking about the program order of a concert. Note the question asks about the first person on stage, not first performer. Look for the part of the poster that indicates the sequence of events.

Steps 1 and 3: The announcement is divided into different sections. Look for the parts of the poster that indicate the sequence of events. At the top is the name of the event and the information that it's free. Then a section marked "When" states the date and time of the event. Following that is information about the location and, finally, who will be speaking or performing.

Step 4: The "kickoff" is a welcome speech by the mayor, so predict that the mayor appears on stage first.

Step 5: Choice **(C)** matches your prediction and is correct; a welcome speech kicking off the event logically precedes the performances. Choice (A) is incorrect: although the marching band is the first performer listed, it will follow Mayor Edugyan's kickoff address. Choice (B) is also incorrect because the mayor's kickoff precedes all the performances. Finally, choice (D) is incorrect because the poster does provide the information you're asked for.

Details in Graphics

The TEAS also tests your ability to identify relevant information presented in graphical form such as maps, graphs, charts, or illustrations. TEAS questions might require you to read examples of graphical representation, recognize figures and graphics within a piece of text, or determine relationships between visual elements.

Study this example of how an expert would approach a question accompanied by an information-laden graphic:

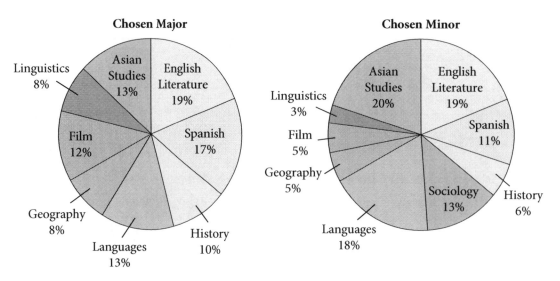

Total students = 500

Brockmeier Liberal Arts College Student Survey Results

Question	Analysis
At Brockmeier College, students do not major and minor in the same field. According to the charts, what percentage of Brockmeier College students choose Film as their major or as a minor field of study?	**Step 2:** The question asks for the total percentage of students who choose Film as a major or minor.
	Steps 1 and 3: The two charts provide data from a survey of 500 students—specifically percentages of students in each major (left) and minor (right). Because the question asks about majors and minors, look at both pie charts and read the percentages from the Film "slice."
	Step 4: Because students never major and minor in the same field, the percentages can be added: 12% report Film as their major, while another 5% report it as their minor. Add: $12 + 5 = 17$.
(A) 5	**Step 5:** This is the percentage of Film minors.
(B) 12	This is the percentage of Film majors.
(C) 17	Correct. This matches your prediction.
(D) 85	If you calculated the number of students with Film as a major or minor, then you would get 85. However, the question asks for the percentage, and percentages are directly stated in the charts.

KEY IDEAS

- Read each question stem carefully so you know exactly what it is asking.
- When researching the answer to a detail question, don't get distracted by extraneous information.
- Pay attention to headings and labels in graphics so you know the location of key information.

Reading for Details Practice Questions

Questions 1–2 refer to this passage.

Most life is fundamentally dependent on photosynthetic organisms that store radiant energy from the Sun. In almost all the world's ecosystems and food chains, photosynthetic organisms such as plants and algae are eaten by other organisms, which are then consumed by still others. The existence of organisms that are not dependent on the Sun's light has long been established, but until recently they were regarded as anomalies.

Over the last 20 years, however, research in deep-sea areas has revealed the existence of entire ecosystems in which the primary producers are chemosynthetic bacteria that are dependent on energy from within the Earth itself. Indeed, growing evidence suggests that these sub-sea ecosystems model the way in which life first came about on this planet.

1. The passage states that most life depends ultimately on which of the following?

   (A) Photosynthetic plants and algae
   (B) Sub-sea ecosystems
   (C) Chemosynthetic bacteria
   (D) Sunlight

2. According to the passage, which of the following statements is true about both photosynthetic and chemosynthetic organisms?

   (A) Both are at the base of their respective food chains.
   (B) Both are capable of receiving energy from the Earth.
   (C) Sunlight is the basic source of energy for both.
   (D) Chemosynthetic organisms are more abundant than photosynthetic organisms.

Questions 3–4 refer to the following timeline.

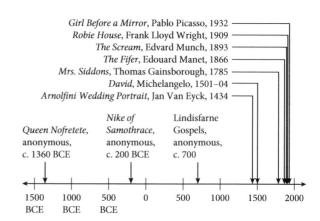

3. How many works of art predate the Common Era?

   (A) 1
   (B) 2
   (C) 3
   (D) 8

4. Which pair of artworks have creation dates that are furthest apart?

   (A) *Nike of Samothrace* and Lindisfarne Gospels
   (B) *Arnolfini Wedding Portrait* and *Mrs. Siddons*
   (C) *The Scream* and *Robie House*
   (D) *Robie House* and *Girl Before a Mirror*

Questions 5–6 refer to the following map.

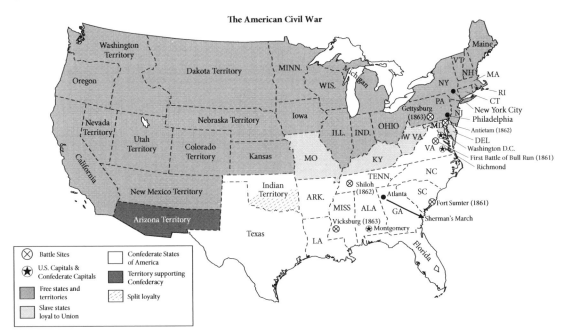

5. Which battlefield site shown is furthest north?

    (A) First Battle of Bull Run
    (B) Shiloh
    (C) Antietam
    (D) Gettysburg

6. Which of the following slave states did NOT join the Confederacy?

    (A) Texas
    (B) Arizona
    (C) West Virginia
    (D) Ohio

Review your work using the explanations in Part Six of this book.

LESSON 3

Making Inferences

LEARNING OBJECTIVES

- Make logical inferences from statements in a stimulus or question stem
- Apply knowledge of inferences to identify and eliminate false and unsupported conclusions

The TEAS will often ask questions about facts or beliefs that are suggested or implied, but not actually stated outright in the passage. These require you to make correct **inferences** based on the provided information and common knowledge. For example, if you saw a person put on a raincoat before heading outside, you would probably infer that it was either raining or expected to rain, even though no one has said anything about the weather.

There are two main requirements for any inference. First, it has to logically follow from the information that's given. An inference is either logically necessary or very likely to be true based on the information given and common sense. Second, inferences are always unstated. When a fact is stated explicitly, it does not need to be inferred.

Incorrect answer choices to inference questions can be eliminated when they contradict the passage, contradict facts that can be inferred from the passage, are contrary to common sense and general knowledge, or are not implied or suggested by the passage at all.

Follow along as a TEAS expert maps a passage and answers two inference questions.

Dear Applicant,

Thank you for applying to our recent job advertisement. We've been rated one of the best companies to work for as well as one of the top companies in our industry. We believe that success is due to the people who work here. Each of our employees has the right skill set for their role and is the best possible fit for their team. We want to maintain the high-functioning ability of our teams. Therefore, we consider each new team member's application with great care.

You can be confident that your qualifications will be given the same thoughtful consideration we give to those of all prospective new employees. This is often the slowest step of the hiring process, and we would appreciate your not calling us during this period for updates on your application. If you have not heard from us within 15 business days of receiving this letter, then we wish you good luck in your job search and invite you to reach out to us about future opportunities.

Question	Analysis
	Step 1: Paragraph 1 establishes that this is a letter acknowledging receipt of a job application. It provides information about the company's goals and how they influence the hiring process. Paragraph 2 explains that the applicant may hear back within 15 business days, but if not, encourages them to apply again.

Question	Analysis
If the job applicant who received the letter above does not hear anything further after one month, what conclusion should she draw?	**Step 2:** This is an inference question. Consider both paragraphs, but especially the second, as well as the information given in the question.
	Step 3: Paragraph 2 explains whether and when an applicant can expect to hear back. The response should come, if at all, within 15 days.
	Step 4: It can be clearly inferred that a person who does not hear from the company within 15 days has not been selected for an interview (if they were, there would be no reason to wish the applicant luck or encourage them to apply for future openings). It can also be inferred that the company does not think the applicants it declines to interview are among the top choices (paragraph 1). Predict that this applicant was not selected to be interviewed.
(A) The company misplaced her contact information.	**Step 5:** This choice is contradicted by the fact that the company has already sent her a letter acknowledging her application.
(B) The hiring manager did not feel she was likely to be the best fit for the role or team.	Correct. This is a good match for the prediction.
(C) The company has not yet determined whom to interview.	The statement in paragraph 2 implies the company does not take more than 15 business days to contact interviewees. Eliminate.
(D) The company is leaning toward hiring someone else but is not ready to rule her out.	There is no support for this. It can be inferred from paragraph 2 that anyone not selected for an interview will remain uncontacted without being explicitly told they were rejected, so the lack of contact does not imply a final decision is still pending.

Here is another inference question on the same passage.

Question	Analysis
Based on the letter, which of the following can be concluded about the company?	**Step 2:** This is an inference question.
	Step 3: The question stem does not point to a particular part of the passage. Review your passage map so you have the letter writer's important points in mind.
	Step 4: Predict the correct answer will be supported by information in the passage.

Question	Analysis
(A) The company expects a large number of applicants for the positions it advertises.	**Step 5:** The first paragraph mentions the job was advertised, so the company has potentially reached a large number of job seekers. This is a generic form letter that doesn't even mention the applicant's name. The letter also implies that applicants should expect to hear back within 15 business days or not at all. It's reasonable to assume from these facts that the company is trying to minimize the amount of time spent communicating with each applicant, which makes sense when there is a large number of applicants. Choice **(A)** is therefore a well-supported conclusion.
(B) The company is fairly small.	Nothing in the passage implies this answer choice is true.
(C) The company has low standards for its employees.	This is directly contradicted in the first paragraph.
(D) The company is brand new.	There is nothing in the passage to support this answer choice. In fact, the statement that the company and its employees are the best implies some history of performance.

Now practice answering some inference questions on your own. After reading and mapping the passage and answering the question, check your work against the explanation that follows.

Packaging on many popular foods is deceiving to consumers. Too often, the print is small and hard to read. Even if you can read it, it's often confusing or intentionally vague. This is especially true on the nutrition label. Consumer protection advocates say the government ought to do something about the nutrition labels on food because the existing laws don't go far enough.

One recent example of legislation that would have addressed these concerns is a bill, which unfortunately died in committee, that would have forced American distributors to include information related to hormones and antibiotics in meat. There is no ingredient list on a package of ground beef to tell consumers what chemicals they may be ingesting, and perhaps there won't be for some time. But don't consumers have a right to information about what they're putting in their bodies?

The author of the passage would probably support which of the following?

(A) A ban on magazine advertisements for cigarettes
(B) Unsolicited grocery store flyers
(C) Fine print on a contract
(D) Allergy information prominently listed on food labels

Explanation

Step 1:

Topic: Incorrect/dishonest food package labels
Scope: Why the gov't should do more to protect consumers
Purpose: To argue for more gov't regulation
¶ 1: Why food labels are bad; advocates say gov't should do something
¶ 2: Example of law author supports—info on hormones/antibiotics in meat; law failed
Author: Such laws are needed

Step 2: The words "probably support" make this an inference question.

Step 3: Your map tells you the author's overall position on the topic and says it's in paragraph 2. For confirmation, you could look at the rhetorical question at the end of the passage.

Step 4: Predict that the author would most likely support greater information about food content being made available to consumers.

Step 5: Match your prediction with correct answer **(D)**. The author does not take a position on advertisements of unhealthy products, so it cannot be concluded that the author would support choice (A). Choice (B) is unrelated to the main argument of the passage, which is about food labels, while choice (C) is something the the author would likely be against, based on the complaint about hard-to-read ingredient lists.

> Based on the passage, it is reasonable to assume that
>
> (A) food label laws are primarily an American issue.
> (B) nutrition is not a top priority for the average consumer.
> (C) most companies do not voluntarily provide clear and accurate information on food labels.
> (D) the government has only recently begun to regulate the food industry.

Explanation

Step 2: The words "Based on the passage" and "reasonable to assume that" tell you this is an inference question.

Step 3: The question does not focus on a specific part of the passage, so answer choices need to be checked and eliminated one at a time. Review your passage map so you have the letter writer's important points in mind.

Step 4: The correct answer choice will be a valid inference from the passage.

Step 5: Match your prediction to answer choice **(C)**. It can be inferred from the statement that "existing laws don't go far enough" that a majority of companies in the food industry do not provide more information than legally required. None of the other answer choices are directly contradicted in the passage, but neither are they implied.

KEY IDEAS

- Recognize key terms that signal inference questions.
- Predict what ideas an author would agree with by using the author's statements to infer a logical conclusion.
- Evaluate answer choices by checking whether they logically follow from the passage; eliminate choices that are not fully supported.

Making Inferences Practice Questions

Questions 1–5 refer to the following passage.

In the dog days of summer, there's a difficult choice to make: tripping over a collection of noisy, bulky fans or running up the electric bill with pricey air-conditioning. But at least it's a choice. In the winter months, high heating bills seem to be simply a fact of life. But there is an alternative: the Arizona Desert product line. It's no longer necessary to choose between economy and comfort. You can have both.

On cold nights, lower your thermostat and plug in the time-tested Arizona Desert electric blanket, which *Consumer Services* magazine calls "the most reliable and best value available by a wide margin." Enjoy your coffee on those chilly mornings in our newest product, the Arizona Desert heated robe. Like our blanket, this robe, the first of its kind, contains our patented heating system with an unobtrusive motor that is as silent as it is invisible. Heating coils warm a fluid, which is then circulated by the motor through tubes sewn into the tough but soft insulating fabric. The temperature can be adjusted to within one degree, and the robe or blanket heats up in minutes.

The tough tubing keeps the heated fluid, with our patented chemical formula, completely sealed. It never needs to be replaced, so you are never exposed to any risk of contact with it. If the tubing cracks or tears, or the motor fails, just bring the product immediately to your nearest supplier and get a replacement—no questions asked. Do not try to repair or replace any parts yourself. Using a mere 100 watts for the blanket and 75 watts for the robe (less than the average toaster uses), these products will run for less than 15 cents per day. This is a heating solution that pays for itself, and then pays you.

1. The above passage is most likely excerpted from

   (A) an advertising brochure.
   (B) a consumer reporting magazine.
   (C) a government report.
   (D) a personal email from a close friend.

2. The final paragraph implies that

   (A) the Arizona Desert products are a viable alternative to a standard toaster.
   (B) consumers who use Arizona Desert products will lower their heating costs.
   (C) toasters contribute a major portion of the average household energy budget.
   (D) cost is not a major factor in determining approaches to heating.

3. From the passage, the reader can determine that

   (A) electric blankets are more expensive to purchase than central heating.
   (B) air conditioners use more energy than fans.
   (C) the Arizona Desert company is a new start-up.
   (D) electric blankets are used primarily by those without central heating.

4. Which of the following would the passage's author likely consider least important to a person thinking of purchasing an electric blanket or robe?

   (A) Energy savings
   (B) Safety
   (C) Comfort
   (D) Country of manufacture

5. The warning label on the blanket would likely NOT include which of the following statements?

   (A) Warning! Chemical fluid—toxic!
   (B) Avoid submerging in water, as electric shock could occur.
   (C) Choking hazard—do not swallow.
   (D) Do not disassemble or modify any part of the heating mechanism.

Review your work using the explanations in Part Six of this book.

K

LESSON 4

Understanding Sequences of Events

LEARNING OBJECTIVES

- Identify key words and phrases that denote order and steps
- Apply an understanding of the relationship of events or steps in a sequence to answer a question
- Follow a set of instructions to achieve a result

Series of Events or Actions

When the TEAS presents a stimulus that focuses on the order of events or actions, it is vital to identify the words that tell you in what order to perform the steps or how events happened in relation to each other. To tackle such passages, timelines, or other figures, look for certain key words and phrases.

Sequence and timing key words and phrases place steps chronologically. Here are some examples: *first, second, third*; *before, after, next, finally, later*; *by the time, when/once* [something has happened]; *in the mid-1990s, after the turn of the century.*

Continuation key words may indicate that one step or event is over and the next is beginning. Examples include *moreover, furthermore, also,* and *in addition.*

Following directions requires you to read carefully, noting what materials are needed and what to do with them. A series of actions may be described out of order, as in this example:

> Until the customer has completed the purchase, be available to answer questions.

Here, being available to answer questions happens first, before the customer finishes the purchase. This order of events is indicated by the key word "Until." When a stimulus involves a number of steps given out of order, jotting them down in order may help you keep them straight.

Here are the directions for making tea. Follow along as a TEAS expert answers a question about the sequence of steps.

Question	Analysis
Before boiling water to make tea, make sure you have tea bags ready. Fill a kettle with water and put it on the stove over medium to high heat. While the water is warming, take out the cups you will use. After the water reaches a boil, turn off the heat and pour some into each cup. Finally, add the tea bags.	**Steps 1 and 3:** The paragraph lists the steps to making tea. Note the words "Before," "while," "after," and "finally." These tell you the correct order. Look for "tea bags" to determine where they come in the process. The tea bags appear twice, once at the beginning (when you get them ready) and again at the end (when you add them). It's the latter action that this question mentions, so back up one step from there.

Question	Analysis
The step prior to placing tea bags in the cups is	**Step 2:** This question asks you to correctly identify a particular step in a process.
	Step 4: Predict that the step prior to adding tea bags is pouring water into the cups.
(A) taking out the cups.	**Step 5:** This step is done while the water is heating. Eliminate.
(B) getting the tea bags ready.	This is the first step in the process. Eliminate.
(C) pouring water into the cups.	Correct. This matches your prediction; it's the step immediately before adding tea bags.
(D) putting the water on to boil.	This is part of the second step, after getting the tea bags ready; eliminate.

Following Instructions

The TEAS may give you a set of instructions and ask you to follow them. Then you must find an answer choice that matches the result. Here's an example of how an expert would tackle this kind of question.

Question	Analysis
Start with the list of letters below. Follow the directions to change the list. a d e h n o 1. Reorder the list of letters above by placing the vowels in alphabetical order followed by the consonants in reverse alphabetical order. 2. If a letter is a consonant, add the vowel that comes after it in the alphabet directly after it in the list. 3. If a letter is a vowel, add the consonant that comes after it in the alphabet directly after it in the list.	**Steps 1 and 3:** There are six letters, three vowels and three consonants, and the letters are in alphabetical order. The instructions ask you to (1) reorder the letters, (2) add vowels to the list after the consonants, and (3) add consonants to the list after the vowels.
After step 3, which letter is in the middle of the list?	**Step 2:** This question asks you to reorder a list of letters by following a set of instructions.

Question	Analysis
	Step 4: Follow the instructions, step-by-step. 1. a e o n h d 2. a e o n *o* h *i* d *e* 3. a *b* e *f* o p n o p h i j d e *f* Note that in (2), you insert the vowels after the consonants in the rearranged list, the list that is the output of (1). Then in (3), you insert the consonants in the list that is the output of (2). There are now 15 letters in the list. Count in from both ends to find the middle letter. It is the 8th letter, with 7 letters on either side. a b e f o p n **o** p h i j d e f
(A) h (B) n (C) o (D) p	**Step 5:** The correct answer is **(C)**. After the list has been rearranged and added to according to the instructions, *o* is in the middle of the list.

KEY IDEAS

- When reading a stimulus, note key words and phrases that indicate sequence and time.
- If events or steps are given out of order, construct the proper order mentally or by jotting some notes.
- When following instructions, work step-by-step, making sure to apply the instructions in one step to the result of the previous one.

Understanding Sequences of Events Practice Questions

Questions 1–4 are based on the following instructions.

Creating an Ikebana Floral Arrangement

Materials:

- Shallow dish
- Floral "frog" (disc with short spikes that hold flowers in place)
- Flowers, stems, and other plant material in at least three different lengths

Instructions:

First, fill the dish with 1½ inches of water. Then, place the frog in the dish at the 7:00 position. Put the longest stem at the 11:00 position on the frog. Next, place the second-longest stem on the frog at the 8:00 position, then place the third-longest stem in the 4:00 position.* Now, continue placing all other plant material in any position that pleases you.

*Lean the first three stems toward the right.

1. Based on the information in the steps, where is the third-longest stem placed?

   (A) At the 4:00 position
   (B) At the 8:00 position
   (C) At the 11:00 position
   (D) At any pleasing position

2. The first step in making an ikebana arrangement is

   (A) placing the frog.
   (B) using all plant material.
   (C) adding water to the dish.
   (D) placing the longest stem in the frog.

3. Suppose a florist has four items: a bamboo stem of 4 inches, a chrysanthemum of 5½ inches, an iris of 3 inches, and a pine branch of 8 inches. According to the directions, in what order would the florist place the plants in the frog?

   (A) pine, iris, chrysanthemum, bamboo
   (B) iris, bamboo, chrysanthemum, pine
   (C) pine, chrysanthemum, bamboo, iris
   (D) bamboo, pine, chrysanthemum, iris

4. After the third-longest stem, all other stems should be placed

   (A) in any place.
   (B) at the left.
   (C) at the right.
   (D) in the center.

Questions 5–8 refer to the following passage.

Construction of the Golden Gate Bridge, connecting San Francisco with Marin County, was started in 1933 and finished in 1937. At the time, it was the longest suspension bridge in the world at 4,200 feet, though it lost this title when the Verrazano-Narrows bridge was built in New York in 1964. On the Golden Gate's first day, May 27, only one person was allowed to walk across the bridge, but the next day 200,000 people walked across it. Currently pedestrians can walk the bridge until 6:00 PM Pacific Standard Time, but skateboards, roller skates, and electric scooters are not allowed at any time. Cars, however, cross at all times, at a rate of approximately 112,000 vehicles per day, having paid a toll only in the southbound direction toward San Francisco.

5. If a person wanted to cross the bridge at 8:00 PM Pacific Standard Time, he or she would need to do so

   (A) on an electric scooter.
   (B) in a car.
   (C) on a skateboard.
   (D) on foot.

6. The Golden Gate Bridge was the longest suspension bridge in the world until

   (A) 1934.
   (B) 1944.
   (C) 1954.
   (D) 1964.

7. On May 28, 1937, how many pedestrians crossed the bridge?

   (A) 1
   (B) 4,200
   (C) 112,000
   (D) 200,000

8. In 1936, the Golden Gate bridge was

   (A) begun.
   (B) finished.
   (C) open.
   (D) under construction.

9. Start with the numbered squares below. Follow the directions to rearrange them.

1	2	3	4	5	6	7	8
9	10	11	12	13	14	15	16

   1. Make a larger square out of the first four even-numbered squares, placing the lowest-numbered square in the upper left corner and placing the squares from least to greatest in clockwise fashion.
   2. In the same manner as in step 1, make a larger square from the first four odd-numbered squares.
   3. In the same manner as in step 1, make a larger square from the remaining even-numbered squares.
   4. In the same manner as in step 1, make a larger square from the remaining odd-numbered squares.
   5. Using the 4 × 4 squares created in steps 1–4, make a larger square. Place the square containing the single largest number in the upper left and proceed counterclockwise, each time selecting the remaining 4 × 4 square containing the largest number.

   Which of the following statements is true regarding the result of steps 1–5 above?

   (A) The square numbered 15 is to the right of the square numbered 6.
   (B) The square numbered 10 is above the square numbered 15.
   (C) The square numbered 2 is to the left of the square numbered 12.
   (D) The square numbered 6 is below the square numbered 15.

Review your work using the explanations in Part Six of this book.

Review and Reflect

Think about the questions you answered in these lessons.

- Were you able to approach each question systematically, using the Kaplan Method for Reading?
- Were you able to read the passage strategically, using key words to find important facts and ideas? Did you take brief notes as needed to map the passage?
- Did you feel confident that you understood what the question was asking you to do?
- How well were you able to predict an answer before looking at the answer choices?
- Could you match your prediction to the correct answer?
- If you missed any questions, do you understand why the answer you chose is incorrect and why the right answer is correct? Could you do the question again now and get it right?

Use your thoughts about these questions to guide how you continue to prepare for the TEAS. If you feel you need more review and practice with reading for main ideas and details and making inferences, you should study this chapter some more and use the online Qbank that comes with this book. After you have registered your book at **kaptest.com/booksonline**, log in to your student homepage at **kaptest.com** to use your Qbank.

The TEAS also tests two other areas of *Reading*:

- Passage Structure and Word Choices
- Integrating Ideas to Draw Conclusions

Chapters with lessons addressing these concepts and skills will be included in Kaplan's *ATI TEAS® Strategies, Practice, & Review with 2 Practice Tests*, which will be available for purchase in January 2017.

Mathematics

As a nursing or health science program student, and later in your career as a healthcare professional, you will need to interpret data, perform calculations, and translate real-world situations into math to respond appropriately. You might be reading test results presented as numbers or a graph, calculating medication dosages, interpreting research study results, or planning patient care. The TEAS *Mathematics* content area tests your ability to perform arithmetic and algebra. You will apply these skills to solving word problems; interpreting charts and graphs; using descriptive statistics to characterize data sets; understanding relationships between numbers; calculating geometric values; and using measurements appropriately, including by converting from one unit of measure to another.

Questions by Content Area

English and language usage 17%

Reading 31%

Science 31%

Mathematics 21%

The TEAS Mathematics Content Area

Of the 170 items on the TEAS, 36 will be in the *Mathematics* content area, and you will have 54 minutes to answer them. Thus, you will have 54 minutes ÷ 36 questions = 1.5 minutes per question.

Of the 36 *Mathematics* questions, 32 will be scored and 4 will be unscored. You won't know which questions are unscored, so do your best on every question.

The 32 scored *Mathematics* questions come from two sub-content areas:

Sub-content Areas	# of Questions
Number and algebra	23
Measurement and data	9

Kaplan's *High-Yield Practice for the New ATI TEAS*® includes a chapter covering the area of *Mathematics* the TEAS tests most:

- Chapter 1: Arithmetic and Algebra

The Kaplan Method for Mathematics

Approaching every *Mathematics* question on the TEAS in a systematic way will help you solve efficiently.

KAPLAN METHOD FOR MATHEMATICS

Step 1: Analyze the information provided.

Step 2: Approach strategically.

Step 3: Evaluate the answer choices.

Step 4: Confirm your answer.

Step 1: Analyze the information provided.

Every TEAS *Mathematics* question will give you the information you need to solve it. This information may be in the question and/or in a table, figure, or other information supplied above the question. The answer choices may also provide useful information, so analyze those as well.

Step 2: Approach strategically.

Unlike a math class, which focuses on a single subject such as algebra, the TEAS tests many types of math. When you look at a new question, pause briefly—give yourself the time it takes to take a deep breath—and think about what type of math you will use to solve. Is the question testing arithmetic? Algebra? Geometry? Call to mind the math rules you use to solve this type of question.

In addition, make sure that you have clearly stated in your mind what you are solving for. It's a shame to do all the math right only to choose the wrong answer because you solved for x when the question was asking for $x - 2$, or because you solved for a possible solution when the question asked for a value that *cannot* be a solution. Make sure you are solving for the right thing.

Finally, use the answer choices to your advantage. For example, if there are two negative numbers and two positive numbers in the answers, then if you can quickly determine that the answer must be negative (or must be positive), you can immediately rule out two choices. If the values in the answers are far apart, then estimating an approximate value may be an efficient approach. If you can tell that the answer must be a little less than 1, and only one answer choice fits that description, then you can choose that answer without doing any calculations.

Step 3: Evaluate the answer choices.

Choose the correct answer from the answer choices. If no choice matches the value you arrived at, then revisit Steps 1 and 2 to see if you overlooked any information or made an error in solving.

Step 4: Confirm your answer.

You're not done yet! Double-check that you've answered the right question. For example, you don't want to choose the time it takes to load one truck if the question asks for the time to load two trucks. Also, make sure your answer makes sense. For example, if a coat cost $100 and it's now on sale, the sale price should be less, not more, than $100.

ARITHMETIC AND ALGEBRA

LEARNING OBJECTIVES

- Perform operations with rational numbers, including fractions, decimals, and percentages
- Isolate and calculate the value of a variable
- Translate word problems into math and solve for an unknown value
- Determine a value using a proportion and calculate percent change and rate of change
- Convert measurements between different metric units
- Use rounding and estimating to solve problems efficiently

Of the 32 scored *Mathematics* questions, 23 (72%) will be in the sub-content area of *Number and algebra*. With these questions, the TEAS tests your ability to use arithmetic and algebra to solve questions presented with numbers, variables, and words. Some questions will concern percentages, proportions, and rates. In addition, you'll solve some questions more easily by using estimation and rounding than by calculating an exact value.

This chapter addresses these skills in five lessons:

Lesson 1: Arithmetic

Lesson 2: Algebra

Lesson 3: Solving Word Problems

Lesson 4: Ratios, Percentages, and Proportions

Lesson 5: Estimating and Rounding

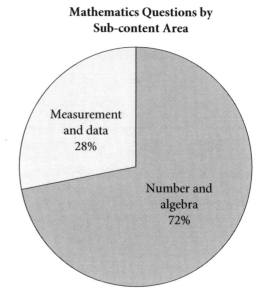

Mathematics Questions by Sub-content Area

Measurement and data 28%

Number and algebra 72%

LESSON 1

Arithmetic

LEARNING OBJECTIVES

- Compare and order rational numbers
- Convert among non-negative fractions, decimals, and percentages
- Perform arithmetic operations with rational numbers

Place Value and the Number Line

The value of a digit (the digits are the integers 0–9) depends on its place or position in the number. This is the **place value**. In this place value chart, which shows the number 679.32815, the digit on the left (6) has the greatest value.

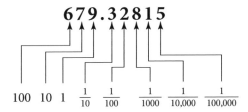

$$679.32815$$

$$100 \quad 10 \quad 1 \quad \frac{1}{10} \quad \frac{1}{100} \quad \frac{1}{1000} \quad \frac{1}{10,000} \quad \frac{1}{100,000}$$

To order numbers, align the place values of the numbers being compared. Start at the left and compare the value of the first digit of each number. Here is how an expert would answer a question about place value.

Question	Analysis
Place the numbers 253, 87, and 216 in order from least to greatest.	**Step 1:** You are given three numbers and asked to put them in order from least to greatest.
(A) 87, 253, 216 (B) 253, 216, 87 (C) 216, 253, 87 (D) 87, 216, 253	**Step 2:** Compare using a place values chart. <table><tr><td>Hundreds</td><td>Tens</td><td>Ones</td></tr><tr><td>2</td><td>5</td><td>3</td></tr><tr><td>0</td><td>8</td><td>7</td></tr><tr><td>2</td><td>1</td><td>6</td></tr></table> The least (smallest) number is the one whose leftmost digit has the smallest place value. This is 87. Now compare the first digit of the remaining numbers. Both numbers have the same digit in the hundreds place, so compare the digits in the tens place. Because 1 is less than 5, 216 is less than 253.

Question	Analysis
	Step 3: The correct answer is **(D)**.
	Step 4: Double-check that you made valid, accurate comparisons and you ordered the numbers as asked. Choice (B) is a trap; the numbers are ordered greatest to least.

You can also use a **number line** to compare numbers. Beginning with zero, numbers increase in value to the right (0, 1, 2, 3, . . .) and decrease in value to the left (−3, −2, −1, 0, . . .). The order in which numbers are placed on the number line will determine which are greater and which are less than other numbers.

A **signed number** tells you two things: the sign tells you the direction from zero, and the number tells you the distance from zero. For example, −3 is three spaces to the left of zero, and +5 is five spaces to the right of zero.

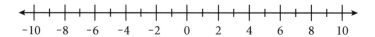

Try this question.

What is the correct order of the numbers 2, −10, and −4, from least to greatest?

(A)   2, −4, −10
(B)   −4, −10, 2
(C)   −10, −4, 2
(D)   2, −10 −4

Explanation

Step 1: You are given three numbers and asked to put them in correct order, from least to greatest.

Step 2: Compare the numbers: −10 lies ten spaces to the left of zero, −4 lies four spaces to the left of zero, and 2 lies two spaces to the right of zero.

Step 3: The correct answer choice is **(C)**.

Step 4: Double-check that you made accurate comparisons and ordered the numbers as asked. Choice (A) is a trap; the digits 2, 4, and 10 are in order from least to greatest, but when the signs are taken into account, the numbers are in order from greatest to least.

Operations With Positive and Negative Numbers

Use a number line to help add signed numbers. For example:

$2 + (−5) = −3$ Begin at +2; move 5 steps in the negative direction (left); end at −3.

$−3 + (−4) = −7$ Begin at −3; move 4 steps in the negative direction (left); end at −7.

To add without a number line, follow these steps:

- If numbers have like signs, add the numbers and keep the same sign.
- If the numbers have different signs, find the difference between the two numbers and write the difference (the answer) with the sign of the larger number.

For example, add $2 + (-5)$. Because the numbers have different signs, subtract: $5 - 2 = 3$. Then use the sign from the larger number—here that's the negative sign with the 5—to get -3.

You can rewrite a subtraction problem as an addition problem. Change the operation symbol to addition and change the sign on the number you are subtracting. Then apply the rules for adding signed numbers.

Here is how the TEAS would ask about operations with positive and negative numbers. See if you can answer this one.

$$-22 + (-13) - (-11) + 27 = ?$$

    (A) -19
    (B)   3
    (C)   7
    (D)   73

Explanation

Step 1: You are given an expression that involves the addition and subtraction of numbers with unlike signs and asked to find its value.

Step 2: Rewrite the subtraction as addition and change the sign of the following number:
$-22 + (-13) + 11 + 27$.
Add the positive terms: $11 + 27 = 38$.
Add the negative terms: $22 + 13 = -35$.
Combine the result: $38 + (-35) = 3$.

Step 3: The correct answer is **(B)**.

Step 4: Double-check your arithmetic, making sure you handled each sign correctly, including when adding numbers with mixed signs in the final step.

Multiplying and dividing signed numbers is no different from other multiplication and division, except that you need to determine whether the solution will be positive or negative. Count the number of negative numbers. If the number of negatives is odd, the answer will be negative. If you have an even number of negative numbers, the answer will be positive.

So for example, to multiply $6(-3)(2)$, first multiply the numbers only: $6 \times 3 \times 2 = 36$. Then, because there is one negative term, the answer is negative: $6(-3)(2) = -36$.

Now you try this example:

$$-(5)(5)(-1)(-3)(2) =$$

    (A) -150
    (B) -2
    (C)   16
    (D)   150

Explanation

Step 1: You are given an expression that involves multiplying numbers with unlike signs and asked to find its value.

Step 2: Multiply the numbers only: $5 \times 5 \times 1 \times 3 \times 2 = 150$. Now, because there are three negative terms and 3 is an odd number, the product is negative: -150.

Step 3: The correct answer is **(A)**.

Step 4: Double-check that your multiplication is correct and that you counted the number of negative signs accurately. Choice (D) has the correct number but the wrong sign.

Fractions, Decimals, and Percents

Fractions

A **fraction** is part of a whole. The top number, the **numerator**, is the number of parts you are working with. The bottom number, the **denominator**, is the number of equal parts in the whole.

There are eight equal parts in this rectangle. Because three are shaded, $\frac{3}{8}$ of the rectangle is shaded.

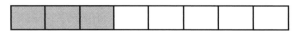

In a **proper fraction**, the numerator is less than the denominator (i.e., $\frac{2}{3}$). A proper fraction represents a quantity less than 1. An **improper fraction** has a numerator with a greater magnitude than that of denominator (i.e., $\frac{9}{8}$). The value is greater than 1. A **mixed number** consists of a whole number and a proper fraction. Its value is greater than 1 (or less than -1 if the improper fraction is negative). Thus, the shaded portion of the following figure represents $\frac{11}{8}$ (written as an improper fraction) or $1\frac{3}{8}$ (written as a mixed number).

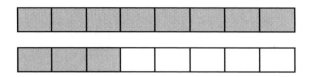

When two fractions have the same denominator, the fraction with the smaller numerator is smaller.

$$\frac{5}{8} < \frac{7}{8}$$

When two fractions have the same numerator, the fraction with the smaller denominator is larger.

$$\frac{5}{6} > \frac{5}{10}$$

When fractions have different numerators and different denominators, a comparison can be difficult. The X method can be used to compare fractions. To compare two positive fractions:

- Draw lines as shown to form an X.
- Multiply denominator × numerator for each line and record the result above each fraction.

$3 \times 4 = 12$ $5 \times 2 = 10$

$$\frac{4}{5} \times \frac{2}{3}$$

The fraction beneath the greater product is the greater fraction. For instance, because $12 > 10$ in the example above, $\frac{4}{5} > \frac{2}{3}$.

Decimals

Decimals are numbers that use place value to show amounts. The number 2.375 is a number between 2 and 3. Read "and" in place of the decimal point. After reading the decimal part, say the place value of the last decimal digit. This number would be read "two and three hundred seventy-five thousandths."

Percentages

Percent means "per hundred" or "out of one hundred." Because percent is a way of showing part of a whole, it has much in common with fractions and decimals. For example, 75% is 0.75 in decimal form. More, 75% can be written as $\frac{75}{100}$, which is $\frac{3}{4}$ when reduced to its simplest form (by dividing the top and bottom of the fraction by 25).

Conversion of Numbers to Different Forms

Percents, fractions, and decimals are all ways to show part of a whole.

Change fractions to decimals by dividing. For example, to express $\frac{3}{8}$ as a decimal, divide 3 by 8: $\frac{3}{8} = 0.375$.

You can change a decimal to a fraction by using place value. For example, to express 0.25 as a fraction, consider that the last digit, 5, is in the hundredths column. So, write 25 over 100 $\left(\frac{25}{100}\right)$. Then reduce by dividing the top and bottom of the fraction by 25: $\frac{25}{100} = \frac{1}{4}$.

Now use your understanding of percents, fractions, and decimals to try two questions on your own.

Express 65% as a fraction in its simplest form.

(A) $\frac{13}{200}$

(B) $\frac{13}{20}$

(C) $\frac{6}{5}$

(D) $6\frac{1}{2}$

Explanation

Step 1: You are given a percent and asked to convert it to a fraction. The answer choices range from tiny, $\frac{13}{200}$, to quite a bit larger, $6\frac{1}{2}$.

Step 2: One way to approach this question is with estimation. If you know that 50% is $\frac{1}{2}$, and you know that 100% is 1, then you know that 65% must be greater than $\frac{1}{2}$ but less than 1. Only one answer choice fits this description.

Another way to solve is through calculating the conversion. Write the percent over 100 and reduce to its simplest form: $65\% = \frac{65}{100} = \frac{13}{20}$.

Step 3: The correct answer is **(B)**.

Step 4: Double-check that you performed the operations accurately and that your answer makes sense. To confirm, you can divide 13 by 20: $\frac{13}{20} = 0.65 = 65\%$. Choice (A) is a trap for those who divided 65 by 1000.

Arithmetic Operations

Operations With Whole Numbers

Addition, subtraction, multiplication, and division are operations. If there are more than two operations in a single expression, they *must* be performed in a specific manner called the **order of operations**. Use the made-up word PEMDAS to remember the order in which to perform the operations in an expression. PEMDAS stands for:

- <u>P</u>arentheses
- <u>E</u>xponents
- <u>M</u>ultiplication and <u>D</u>ivision (from left to right)
- <u>A</u>ddition and <u>S</u>ubtraction (from left to right)

Write out your calculations step-by-step. Perform each operation one at a time and then simplify before you move on. Here is how you would use PEMDAS to answer a question on the TEAS.

Question	Analysis
What is the value of $(3+4) \times 2 + 6$?	**Step 1:** You are given an expression involving addition and multiplication and asked to find its value.
(A) 15 (B) 17 (C) 20 (D) 56	**Step 2:** Use PEMDAS. $(3 + 4) \times 2 + 6$. Start with parentheses: $7 \times 2 + 6$. Next, multiply: $14 + 6$. Now, add: 20.

Question	Analysis
	Step 3: The correct answer is **(C)**.
	Step 4: Double-check that you performed the operations in the right order and that your calculations are correct. Choice (B) results from disregarding the parentheses and multiplying 4×2 first.

Practice working on PEMDAS with this example.

What is the value of $4 + 6 \times (7 - 2)$?

    (A)   34
    (B)   44
    (C)   50
    (D)   68

Explanation

Step 1: You are given an expression with different operations and asked to find its value.

Step 2: Solve, keeping in mind the order of operations (PEMDAS).

$4 + 6 \times (7 - 2)$
Start with parentheses: $4 + 6 \times 5$
Next, multiply: $4 + 30$
Now, add: 34

Step 3: The correct answer is **(A)**.

Step 4: Did you perform the operations in the correct order and do the arithmetic correctly?

Operations With Fractions

To add or subtract fractions that have the same denominator, just add or subtract the numerators and use the common denominator for the result.

$$\frac{3}{7} + \frac{2}{7} = \frac{3+2}{7} = \frac{5}{7}$$

If the denominators are not the same, then you must find a **common denominator**.

For example, to add $\frac{1}{2}$ and $\frac{1}{3}$, you need equivalent fractions with **common denominators**, which is really just the **least common multiple** (LCM) of the given denominators.

- The multiples of 2 are 2, 4, 6.
- The multiples of 3 are 3, 6.
- The LCM is 6, and the common denominator of $\frac{1}{2}$ and $\frac{1}{3}$ is 6.

For each fraction, multiply the denominator by the other denominator to get the new common denominator. Then, multiply the numerator by the same number (whatever you do to the bottom of a fraction, you must do to the top, and vice versa).

$$\text{Change } \frac{1}{2} : \quad \frac{1}{2} \times \frac{3}{3} = \frac{3}{6}$$

$$\text{Change } \frac{1}{3} : \quad \frac{1}{3} \times \frac{2}{2} = \frac{2}{6}$$

Once you have a common denominator, you can continue with the addition.

$$\frac{1}{2} + \frac{1}{3} = \frac{3}{6} + \frac{2}{6} = \frac{5}{6}$$

Question	Analysis
What is the value of $\frac{1}{3} - \frac{1}{4}$?	**Step 1**: You are given an equation with fractions with different denominators and asked to subtract.
(A) $\frac{7}{12}$ (B) $\frac{1}{7}$ (C) $\frac{1}{12}$ (D) $-\frac{1}{1}$	**Step 2**: The common denominator of $\frac{1}{3}$ and $\frac{1}{4}$ is 12 (the LCM of 3 and 4). $\frac{1}{3} \times \frac{4}{4} = \frac{4}{12} \qquad \frac{1}{4} \times \frac{3}{3} = \frac{3}{12}$ Now you can subtract: $\frac{4}{12} - \frac{3}{12} = \frac{1}{12}$
	Step 3: The correct answer is **(C)**.
	Step 4: Double-check that you correctly multiplied the top and bottom of each fraction and then subtracted the numerators.

To multiply fractions, multiply the numerators straight across and the denominators straight across.

$$\frac{2}{5} \times \frac{2}{3} = \frac{2 \times 2}{5 \times 3} = \frac{4}{15}$$

To divide fractions, multiply the first fraction by the reciprocal (the numerator and denominator change places) of the second fraction.

$$\frac{1}{8} \div \frac{3}{4} = \frac{1}{8} \times \frac{4}{3} = \frac{4}{24}$$

You can first convert mixed numbers to improper fractions by multiplying the denominator by the whole number, adding the numerator to that product, and placing the sum over the denominator.

To convert $2\frac{1}{4}$ to an improper fraction:

- Multiply the whole number part by the denominator of the fraction part: 2×4.
- Add this product to the numerator: $(2 \times 4) + 1$.
- Record this result as the numerator: $(2 \times 4) + 1$.
- Keep the denominator the same as in the fraction part: $\dfrac{(2 \times 4) + 1}{4}$.
- Simplify: $2\frac{1}{4} = \dfrac{(2 \times 4) + 1}{4} = \dfrac{8 + 1}{4} = \dfrac{9}{4}$.

Practice using mixed numbers with this problem.

What is the value of $2\frac{1}{4} \times 3\frac{2}{3}$, converted to a mixed number?

(A) 1

(B) $\dfrac{15}{12}$

(C) $6\frac{1}{6}$

(D) $8\frac{1}{4}$

Explanation

Step 1: You are given an expression with mixed numbers and asked for its value as a mixed number.

Step 2: Convert the mixed numbers to improper fractions before multiplying the values. The final step is to simplify the equation.

$$2\frac{1}{4} \times 3\frac{2}{3} = \frac{(4 \times 2) + 1}{4} \times \frac{(3 \times 3) + 2}{3} = \frac{9}{4} \times \frac{11}{3} = \frac{99}{12} = 8\frac{3}{12} = 8\frac{1}{4}$$

Step 3: The correct answer is **(D)**.

Step 4: Double-check that your arithmetic is correct and your answer makes sense. Because $2 \times 3 = 6$ and $3 \times 4 = 12$, it makes sense that $2\frac{1}{4} \times 3\frac{2}{3}$ is about halfway between 6 and 12.

KEY IDEAS

- A number line is a tool that helps you compare and order rational numbers.
- Be alert for the effect of negative numbers in multiplication and division.
- Any number can be represented as a fraction, decimal, or percent.
- The key to evaluating an expression is the order of operations (PEMDAS).

Arithmetic Practice Questions

1. Convert 0.32 to a fraction and percent.

    (A) $\frac{4}{25}$, 0.32%

    (B) $\frac{8}{25}$, 3.2%

    (C) $\frac{8}{25}$, 32%

    (D) $\frac{4}{25}$, 32%

2. What is the least common multiple of 4, 8, and 10?

    (A) 10
    (B) 20
    (C) 40
    (D) 80

3. Order the following fractions from least to greatest:
$\frac{3}{8}, \frac{2}{5}, \frac{1}{4}$.

    (A) $\frac{1}{4}, \frac{2}{5}, \frac{3}{8}$

    (B) $\frac{1}{4}, \frac{3}{8}, \frac{2}{5}$

    (C) $\frac{3}{8}, \frac{1}{4}, \frac{2}{5}$

    (D) $\frac{2}{5}, \frac{3}{8}, \frac{1}{4}$

4. What is the sum of $1\frac{5}{8}$ and $\frac{7}{12}$?

    (A) $2\frac{1}{24}$

    (B) $2\frac{5}{24}$

    (C) $2\frac{7}{24}$

    (D) $2\frac{11}{24}$

5. What is the value of $81 + 324 \div 27 - 18 + 17(12)$.

    (A) 143
    (B) 195
    (C) 201
    (D) 279

6. What is the value of $8 + (2 + 5) \times 6$?

    (A) 21
    (B) 40
    (C) 50
    (D) 90

Review your work using the explanations in Part Six of this book.

LESSON 2
Algebra

LEARNING OBJECTIVES

- Recognize a variable in an algebraic expression
- Use the correct arithmetic operations to isolate a variable
- Efficiently calculate the value of a variable

A **variable** is a letter used to represent a numerical value that is unknown. The value of a specific variable (such as x) will be the same throughout a given problem, but it can differ from one problem to another.

A **constant** is a value that doesn't change, typically a number. For example, in the expression $x + 6$, x is the variable and 6 is the constant.

A **term** is a variable, constant, or the product of a constant and a variable. A term containing only a number is called a *constant term* because it contains no variables. The following are all terms: y, 42, and $7a$.

Like terms are terms that can be combined. Simplify algebraic expressions by combining like terms.

Isolating a Variable

The key to solving an equation is to do the same thing to both sides of the equation until you have the variable by itself on one side of the equation and all of the numbers on the other side.

Use **inverse operations** to move terms from the side of the equation containing the variable to the other side. Inverse operations are arithmetic operations that are used to cancel or "undo" each other:

- Addition and subtraction cancel each other.
- Multiplication and division cancel each other.

Here's an example of how an expert combines like terms to simplify an expression.

Question	Analysis
$y + 7 + 3y + 10$ Which of the following is equivalent to the above expression?	**Step 1:** The question gives you an expression containing like terms, constant terms, and terms with the variable y. It asks you to find the equivalent value among the answer choices, which also contain constant terms and terms with y.
(A) $4y + 3$ (B) $2y + 7$ (C) $3y + 70$ (D) $4y + 17$	**Step 2:** Simplify by combining like terms. First, combine y and $3y$: $y + 3y = 4y$. Next, combine 7 and 10: $7 + 10 = 17$. Then, add the unlike terms: $4y + 17$.
	Step 3: The correct answer is choice **(D)**.
	Step 4: Check that you've performed the arithmetic correctly.

Now study how a test expert uses inverse operations to isolate a variable.

Question	Analysis
$x + 6 = 9$ In the above equation, what is the value of x?	**Step 1:** The question presents an equation and asks you to solve for the value of x. In this equation, x is added to 6.
(A) 0 (B) 3 (C) 6 (D) 15	**Step 2:** To get the variable x alone on one side, you must undo the addition with the inverse operation. The inverse of adding 6 is subtracting 6. Therefore, subtracting 6 from the left side of the equation will cancel out the $+6$. Make sure that whatever you do to one side of the equation, you also do to the other, so subtract 6 from both sides: $x + 6 - 6 = 9 - 6$. Next, simplify both sides: $x = 3$.
	Step 3: The correct answer is **(B)**.
	Step 4: Check your answer by plugging it in for x in the original equation: $3 + 6 = 9$.

Now you try a question. This one involves multiplication and division.

$$5a = 20$$

In the above equation, what is the value of a?

(A) 4
(B) 5
(C) 15
(D) 25

Explanation

Step 1: The question asks for the value of a. In this equation, a is multiplied by 5.

Step 2: To get the variable a alone on one side, you must undo the multiplication with the inverse operation. The inverse of multiplying by 5 is dividing by 5, so dividing the left side of the equation by 5 will cancel out the multiplier 5. Whatever you do to one side of the equation, you must also do to the other, so divide by 5 on both sides, then simplify.

$$\frac{5a}{5} = \frac{20}{5}$$
$$a = 4$$

Step 3: The correct answer is **(C)**.

Step 4: Check your answer by plugging it in for a in the original equation: $5 \times 4 = 20$.

Note that a variable sometimes appears on both sides of an equation; however, you'll still use inverse operations to isolate the variable. Try this one.

$$7y + 4 = 3y + 12$$

In the above equation, what is the value of y?

(A) 1.6
(B) 2
(C) 4
(D) 8

Explanation

Step 1: The question asks for the value of y. The variable y appears on both sides of the equation. There is both addition and multiplication on each side.

Step 2: To get the variable y alone on one side, you must undo both the addition and the multiplication with the appropriate inverse operations. Start by subtracting 4 from both sides: $7y + 4 - 4 = 3y + 12 - 4$. And simplify: $7y = 3y + 8$.

Subtract $3y$ from both sides: $7y - 3y = 3y + 8 - 3y$. And simplify: $4y = 8$.

Divide both sides by 4: $y = 2$.

Step 3: The correct answer is **(B)**.

Step 4: Check your answer by plugging it in for y in the original equation.

$$(7 \times 2) + 4 = (3 \times 2) + 12$$
$$14 + 4 = 6 + 12$$
$$18 = 18$$

KEY IDEAS

- Simplify algebraic expressions by combining like terms.
- Use inverse operations to isolate the variable on one side of an equation, with all the numbers on the other side.
- Always do the same thing to both sides of an equation.

Algebra Practice Questions

1. $2x + 16 = 30$

   Solve for x in the equation above. Which of the following is correct?
   (A) 7
   (B) 14
   (C) 23
   (D) 46

2. $5y - 11 + 9y + 81$

   Simplify the expression above. Which of the following is correct?
   (A) $4y - 92$
   (B) $4y + 70$
   (C) $14y + 70$
   (D) $14y + 92$

3. $10b - 21 = 9$

   Solve for b in the equation above. Which of the following is correct?
   (A) -11
   (B) -10
   (C) 3
   (D) 30

4. Find the sum of the expressions $44x - 1$ and $12x + 5$.

   Which of the following is correct?
   (A) $32x + 4$
   (B) $32x - 6$
   (C) $56x - 6$
   (D) $56x + 4$

5. $\dfrac{5a}{2} = 2a + 5$

   Solve for a in the equation above. Which of the following is correct?
   (A) $\dfrac{5}{3}$

   (B) $\dfrac{10}{3}$

   (C) 5
   (D) 10

Review your work using the explanations in Part Six of this book.

LESSON 3

Solving Word Problems

LEARNING OBJECTIVES

- Translate problems described in words into math expressions, equations, and inequalities
- Solve word problems that describe real-world scenarios

Word problems, by definition, require you to translate English into math. Therefore, a key to solving word problems is knowing how to translate various words and phrases into their mathematical equivalents.

The following table lists words and phrases that commonly appear in word problems, along with their mathematical translations.

When you see:	Think:
sum, plus, more than, added to, combined, total	$+$
minus, less than, difference between, decreased by	$-$
is, was, equals, is equivalent to, is the same as, adds up to	$=$
times, product, multiplied by, of, twice, double, triple	$\times$
divided by, quotient, over, per, out of, into	$\div$
what, how many, how much, a number	x, a, etc.

Try translating the following English phrases into the equivalent math.

English   **Math**

1. b is 7 more than a.   _____

2. y is half of x.   _____

3. m decreased by 3 is twice n.   _____

4. Malia earns 20 percent more than Lola.   _____

5. The product of a and b is twice their sum.   _____

6. There are at least three times as many carrots as tomatoes. _____

Now check how you did:

1. $b = a + 7$
2. $y = \dfrac{x}{2}$
3. $m - 3 = 2n$
4. $M = 1.2L$
5. $ab = 2(a + b)$
6. $c \geq 3t$ or $t \leq \dfrac{1}{3}c$

Word problems on the TEAS sometimes include information that is unnecessary to solve the problem. Be sure to distinguish between important and irrelevant information.

See how a test expert uses the relevant information in a word problem to answer this question.

Question	Analysis
Kendra has just purchased an exercise tracker. She also has an app to analyze the data and calculate how many calories she burns. Kendra's step length is 2 feet 3 inches. Which of the following is the distance she will travel if she walks 3500 steps?	**Step 1:** The question provides Kendra's step length and the number of steps she walks, and it asks for the distance she travels. The first two sentences about Kendra's exercise tracker and her app are irrelevant to answering the question.
(A) 3500 feet (B) 7350 feet (C) 7875 feet (D) 8050 feet	**Step 2:** Because the answer choices are given in feet, convert the step length of 2 feet 3 inches into decimal form. Three inches is one-fourth of a foot, or 0.25 feet. Thus, 2 feet 3 inches = 2.25 feet. Next, multiply the length of each step by the number of steps: 2.25 feet × 3500 steps = 7875 feet.
	Step 3: The correct answer is **(C)**.
	Step 4: Check your answer by dividing it by the number of steps: 7875 ÷ 3500 = 2.25. This is the length of each step.

Try this one yourself. Identify the relevant information and translate from English into math.

A medical seminar is being held as part of a yearly science and technology conference. The seminar is attended by a total of 210 doctors, nurses, and scientists. One-fifth of the attendees are nurses, and one-third of the attendees are doctors. How many attendees are neither doctors nor nurses?

(A) 42
(B) 70
(C) 98
(D) 112

Explanation

Step 1: The relevant information is the total number of seminar attendees, the three different types of attendees, and the fraction of the total who are nurses and the fraction of the total who are doctors. You need to find the number of attendees who are not doctors or nurses.

Step 2: First, translate "one-fifth of the attendees are nurses" as $210 \times \dfrac{1}{5} = 42$. There are 42 nurses. Translate "one-third of the attendees are doctors": $210 \times \dfrac{1}{3} = 70$. There are 70 doctors. Therefore, the total number of doctors and nurses is $42 + 70 = 112$. Subtract this from the total attendees to find the number who are neither doctors nor nurses: $210 - 112 = 98$.

Step 3: The correct answer is **(C)**.

Step 4: Check that you applied the correct fractions to the correct groups and that you performed your calculations correctly.

Sometimes, a word problem on the TEAS won't require you to solve for a value. Instead, it will ask you to identify the expression among the answer choices that correctly matches the language in the question stem. Try the following question.

> A dog groomer charges x dollars for each small dog and y dollars for each large dog. Which of the following expressions correctly represents the amount of money the groomer will charge in dollars for three small dogs and two large dogs?
>
> (A) $3x + 2y$
> (B) $5(x + y)$
> (C) $5xy$
> (D) $6(x + y)$

Explanation

Step 1: The question provides the prices the groomer charges for small and large dogs and a variable to represent each, as well as the number of dogs of each size. You're asked to find the expression that represents how much the groomer will charge in the scenario described.

Step 2: Because each small dog is represented by x, and there are three small dogs, multiply x by 3 to yield $3x$. The large dogs are represented by y, and there are two of them, so multiply y by 2 to yield $2y$. Now add the two parts to determine the total: $3x + 2y$.

Step 3: The correct answer is **(A)**. Choice (B) incorrectly combines both prices charged and multiplies by the total number of dogs. Choice (C) incorrectly multiplies the prices and multiplies that product by the total number of dogs. Choice (D) incorrectly combines the two prices and multiplies this sum by the product of the dogs of both sizes.

Step 4: Check your answer by plugging in real dollar values for x and y (for example, $x = 5$ and $y = 10$) and then calculating the total amount the groomer will charge as described in the question stem: $(3 \times \$5) + (2 \times \$10) = \$35$. Now plug $5 for x and $10 for y into the answer choices to see which equals $35.

KEY IDEAS

- Be sure to distinguish between important and unimportant information within word problems.
- Don't be intimidated by lengthy word problems; translate the English into mathematical expressions step-by-step.
- Determine whether you actually need to solve the problem or only identify which mathematical expression it represents.

Solving Word Problems Practice Questions

1. Karina buys lunch at the cafeteria for herself and her son. They both get a soda for $1.50. Karina gets an $8.00 sandwich for herself, and her son has the mac 'n' cheese for $4.75. How much does Karina spend altogether on lunch?

   (A) $12.75
   (B) $14.25
   (C) $15.75
   (D) $28.50

2. Jamal just received a promotion at work, and now he wants to begin saving money. His new salary is $2,875 a month, and his bills come to $2,360 a month. He also wants to have some fun, so he plans to save half of what's left over after paying his bills. How much will he save each month?

   (A) $207.50
   (B) $257.50
   (C) $515.00
   (D) $1030.00

3. A teacher is handing out crayons to students that they will use in an art project, drawing either a landscape scene or a portrait of a family member. Of the students, 9 have chosen to draw a landscape, and 3 have chosen to draw a portrait. The teacher has 60 crayons and wants to distribute them equally. How many crayons should she give each student?

   (A) 5
   (B) 6
   (C) 10
   (D) 20

4. Tyler makes $80 of profit on every six pallets of strawberries he sells at his roadside stand. It takes two bales of straw to grow each pallet of strawberries. How many bales of straw will Tyler need to earn a $400 profit?

   (A) 15
   (B) 30
   (C) 50
   (D) 60

5. Kaitlyn lives 10 miles from her work. Each day, she travels at an average speed of 40 miles per hour to get to work in the morning. In the afternoon, due to heavier traffic, she averages only 30 miles per hour on the trip home. How much time does Kaitlyn spend traveling to and from work each day?

   (A) 30 minutes
   (B) 35 minutes
   (C) 40 minutes
   (D) 1 hour 10 minutes

6. A therapist is considering jobs at two different clinics. Clinic A pays therapists $25 per patient treated plus a flat weekly salary of $200, and each therapist is assigned 30 patients a week. Clinic B pays therapists $40 per patient treated, with no additional salary. What is the minimum number of patients per week the therapist would need to treat at Clinic B to exceed the income he'd make at Clinic A?

   (A) 23
   (B) 24
   (C) 30
   (D) 31

7. A highway on-ramp contains a traffic light to regulate the flow of traffic onto the highway. The light allows one car to pass every 10 seconds, one car to pass every 15 seconds, or one car to pass every 20 seconds, depending on the flow of traffic on the highway. Which of the following expressions represents the number of cars, n, that can pass through this light in 15 minutes, assuming a continuous flow of cars?

   (A) $10 \geq n \geq 20$
   (B) $10 \leq n \leq 20$
   (C) $45 \leq n \geq 90$
   (D) $45 \leq n \leq 90$

8. Each day, 36 gallons of water are applied to a garden. One-fourth of this amount is used to grow vegetables. The water applied to the vegetables must first pass through a filter. The filter can process 360 gallons of water before being replaced, and it is only used to filter the water applied to the vegetables. After how many days will the filter need to be replaced?

   (A) 4
   (B) 10
   (C) 18
   (D) 40

Review your work using the explanations in Part Six of this book.

LESSON 4

Ratios, Percentages, and Proportions

LEARNING OBJECTIVES

- Relate the value of different quantities as a ratio or percentage
- Calculate percentage changes
- Determine the value of an unknown quantity using proportions
- Solve problems using rates

Ratios

Ratios are representations of the relationship of one quantity to another. They can be expressed verbally (for example, "The ratio of cats to dogs is 3 to 4") or by separating the two quantities with a colon (as in 3:4). Ratios can also be written as fractions (e.g., $\frac{3}{4}$). In order to perform calculations using ratios, you will use this format. Because it is common practice to reduce ratios to their lowest terms, ratios do not necessarily specify the actual quantities. For instance, if there were 9 cats and 12 dogs in a pet store, the ratio $\frac{9}{12}$ can be simplified to $\frac{3}{4}$ by dividing both the numerator and denominator by 3.

Ratios can be either "part to part" or **"part to whole."** The example above is a **part-to-part ratio** because it compares cats to dogs. This situation could also be expressed in terms of a **part-to-whole ratio** of cats to total animals. The numerator would still express the number of cats, but the denominator would come from the sum of cats and dogs: $\frac{9}{9+12} = \frac{9}{21}$, which simplifies to $\frac{3}{7}$.

Study how an expert would approach a ratio question.

Question	Analysis
There are 35 staff members at a meeting. Fifteen of the staff members are nurses, and the rest are doctors. What is the ratio of doctors to nurses?	**Step 1:** The question gives the number of staff members and how many of them are nurses, and asks for the ratio of doctors to nurses.
(A) $\frac{3}{7}$ (B) $\frac{3}{4}$ (C) $\frac{4}{3}$ (D) $\frac{7}{3}$	**Step 2:** This question is asking about a part-to-part ratio, doctors:nurses. Determine the number for each of the parts and express the ratio as a fraction. Since there are 35 total staff and 15 are nurses, there are $35 - 15 = 20$ doctors. The ratio of doctors to nurses is thus $\frac{20}{15}$.

Question	Analysis
	Step 3: Although none of the answer choices is $\frac{20}{15}$, choice **(C)** is $\frac{20}{15}$ reduced to its simplest terms.
	Step 4: Be certain you calculated the ratio that was asked for and check your calculations. Choice (B) is the ratio of nurses to doctors.

Percentages

Percentages are the ratio of a quantity to 100. If 4% of the parts made by a factory are defective, then 4 out of every 100 or $\frac{4}{100}$ are defective. It is possible to have values greater than 100%. For instance, this year's sales for a store could be 120% of last year's. As you learned in Lesson 1: Arithmetic, converting between percentages and decimal values is merely a matter of moving the decimal two places to the left when converting from percent to decimal or to the right when converting from decimal to percent. For instance, 27% = 0.27 and 1.13 = 113%.

Test questions and real-world situations may require calculating percentage increase or decrease using the formula $\frac{\text{new amount} - \text{old amount}}{\text{old amount}} \times 100\%$. If the change is a decrease, the result will be negative. Study this example.

Question	Analysis
Jack's doctor increased the dosage of his medication from 80 milligrams to 100 milligrams. What was the percentage increase of the dosage?	**Step 1:** The problem describes an increase from 80 to 100 and asks for the percentage increase.
(A) 20% (B) 25% (C) 80% (D) 125%	**Step 2:** Using the applicable formula, the percent increase is $\frac{100-80}{80} \times 100\%$. This simplifies to $\frac{20}{80} \times 100\%$, which is 25%.
	Step 3: Choice **(B)** is correct.
	Step 4: Check to be certain you answered the correct question and that your calculations are correct. Choice (A) is a typical trap answer since it is 20 ÷ 100 rather than 20 ÷ 80. Choice (D) might be tempting because the new dosage is 125% of the original dosage, but the *increase* is only 25%.

Pay close attention to the exact wording of percentage change questions. Had the question above asked "The new dosage is what percentage of the previous dosage?" the correct answer would have been 125% rather than 25%.

Rates

Rates are ratios with units in the numerator and denominator, such as the price of corn in dollars/bushel or speed measured in kilometers/hour. Ratios can have units as well, but the units in rates have a fixed relationship. The number of cats in the pet store in the ratio example above could be increased without affecting the number of dogs. However, if the number of bushels of corn is increased, then the dollar cost will increase proportionately.

Another way to describe rates is to use the **constant of proportionality**, often represented by the letter k. For instance, if corn costs $4/bushel, then $k = 4$ and the total price of any amount of corn is $k(b)$, where b is the number of bushels.

If it takes 30 minutes for 150 cc of a solution to drip from an IV bag, then the *rate* of infusion is $\dfrac{150 \text{ cc}}{30 \text{ minutes}}$. **Unit rates** are rates that are restated so that the value of the denominator is 1. In this example, that would be $5\dfrac{\text{cc}}{\text{min}}$. Unit rates can be very useful because they show the rate of change of the quantity in the numerator per single unit change in the quantity of the denominator. Try applying this principle in the question below.

> A certain IV solution drips at the rate of $5\dfrac{\text{cc}}{\text{min}}$. If there are 300 cc of solution remaining in the IV bag, how much longer will the bag last, assuming the rate remains constant?
>
> (A)   30 minutes
> (B)   60 minutes
> (C)   300 minutes
> (D)   1500 minutes

Explanation

Step 1: The question provides a drip rate and a quantity and asks how long that quantity would last at the given rate.

Step 2: The bag empties at the rate of $5\dfrac{\text{cc}}{\text{min}}$ and contains 300 cc, so it would take $\dfrac{300}{5} = 60$ minutes to deplete the contents of the bag.

Step 3: Choice **(B)** is correct. Choice (D) is a trap answer obtained by multiplying the rate times the amount of fluid. If the rate were $5\dfrac{\text{cc}}{\text{min}}$ and the solution were dripping for 300 minutes, then a total of 1500 cc would be administered.

Step 4: Check your math and your units. Here, you want to end up with minutes (the unit in the answer choices), and you get that by dividing the cc by cc so those units cancel out, leaving just the minutes: $\text{cc} \div \dfrac{\text{cc}}{\text{min}} = \text{cc} \times \dfrac{\text{min}}{\text{cc}} = \text{min}.$

In complex ratio and rate problems, paying close attention to the units (as was done in Step 4 above) can be the key to determining whether to divide or multiply.

Some rate questions may involve algebra and graphical information displayed on a **coordinate grid**. As shown on the graph with the question below, the coordinate grid is composed of a horizontal *x*-axis and a vertical *y*-axis. The place where they meet is called the origin.

The points on a coordinate grid represent horizontal and vertical distances from the origin. The values increase from left to right on the x-axis and from bottom to top on the y-axis. Negative values of x are to the left of the origin; negative values of y are below the origin. Any point can be located on the coordinate grid by its x and y values, conventionally written as (x, y). The line that passes through any two points on a coordinate grid can be defined by the equation $y = m(x) + b$, where m represents the **slope** of the line and b is the value of y where the line crosses the y-axis. The slope represents the change in the y value per unit change in the x value. Thus, m represents the value of a ratio; if the units of the y and x axes are proportionately related, then m is also a rate.

Study how this information applies to a question.

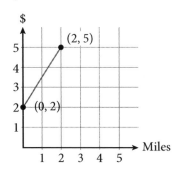

Question	Analysis
If the graph shows the taxi fare in dollars on the y-axis and the miles traveled on the x-axis, and the cost per mile does not vary, what would be the fare for a 10-mile trip?	**Step 1:** The question refers to a line on a coordinate grid showing miles and taxi fares and asks what the fare would be for 10 miles.
(A) $10 (B) $12 (C) $15 (D) $17	**Step 2:** Because the rate will help to answer the question, determine the slope of the line. Compare the two points on the line, (0, 2) and (2, 5). The fare increased by $3 (5 − 2), and the mileage increased by 2 miles (2 − 0). Therefore, the slope is $\frac{3}{2} = 1.50$, and the units are $\frac{\$}{mi}$. The y-intercept on the graph is $2, which is the charge just to get into the taxi. The additional charge to travel 10 miles is $1.50 \times 10 = \$15$ for a total fare of $17.
	Step 3: Choice **(D)** is correct.
	Step 4: Check that you have answered the question that was asked and confirm your calculations.

Proportions

A **proportion** is an equation that sets two ratios equal to each other, for instance, $\dfrac{1}{3}=\dfrac{4}{12}$. Proportions can be used to solve for an unknown quantity when three of the values of a proportion are known, such as when $\dfrac{1}{3}=\dfrac{4}{x}$. The most efficient way to solve proportions is to **cross multiply** the numerator of each ratio by the denominator of the other ratio and set the products equal to each other. For this example, that would be $1 \times x = 3 \times 4$, which simplifies to $x = 12$. Study this example to see how cross multiplying is used in a word question:

Question	Analysis
James has a storage tank to collect rainwater for household use. Unfortunately, there was a severe dry spell where he lives, and the tank ran dry. James added 12 gallons of water to the empty tank, and the gauge on the tank read 5% full. What is the capacity of the tank?	**Step 1:** The problem states that 12 gallons is 5% of the capacity of a tank and asks for the full capacity.

(A) 60 gallons
   (B) 100 gallons
   (C) 120 gallons
   (D) 240 gallons
	Step 2: Set up a proportion to solve this, remembering that a percent is a ratio with 100 in the denominator: $\dfrac{5}{100}=\dfrac{12}{C}$, where C is the capacity of the tank. Each ratio in the proportion represents how "full" the tank is. Cross multiply to obtain $5C = 1200$. Divide both sides by 5, so $C = 240$ gallons.

	Step 3: Choice **(D)** is correct.
	Step 4: Verify that you set up the proportion correctly and check your calculations.

Some questions may ask you to calculate an unknown percentage or to derive a number that is a certain percentage of another number. Proportions are an ideal tool to use to solve such problems. Try this one on your own.

What percent of 5 is 4?

    (A) 4%
    (B) 45%
    (C) 80%
    (D) 125%

Explanation

Step 1: The question asks you to determine what percentage 4 is of 5.

Step 2: Because percent is the ratio of a quantity to 100, you can set up a proportion: $\frac{4}{5} = \frac{x}{100}$. Cross multiply to get $400 = 5x$. Divide both sides by 5 to find that $x = 80$.

Step 3: Choice **(C)** is correct. Notice that you could have answered this question without doing any math. Logic dictates that $\frac{4}{5}$ is greater than $\frac{1}{2}$ but less than 1, so the answer must be between 50% and 100% and **(C)** is the only choice that falls within this range.

Step 4: Double-check that you set up the correct proportion and that your math is correct.

KEY IDEAS

- Ratios show the relationship between two quantities; the values in the ratio may or may not be the actual amounts of the quantities.
- Percentages are ratios that express the number or rate of something per 100 of that thing.
- Percentage change is always calculated relative to the original amount.
- A proportion, which is an equation setting two ratios equal to each other, is a good tool to use with percentage questions.

Ratios, Percentages, and Proportions Practice Questions

1. Juanita made an investment in the stock market. The value of her investment declined by 20%, but then it increased by 50% from that reduced value. What was the overall percent change in the value of her investment?

   (A) 30% decrease
   (B) No change
   (C) 20% increase
   (D) 30% increase

2. Sixty is 15% of what number?

   (A) 180
   (B) 400
   (C) 600
   (D) 900

3. Mary is restocking the inventory of first-aid supplies. The ratio of ointment to bandages to swabs should be maintained at 2:5:8. The current inventory is 6 tubes of ointment, 10 bandages, and 20 swabs. How many of which two types of supplies does she have to add to bring the ratio to its specified value?

   (A) 5 bandages and 4 swabs
   (B) 2 tubes of ointment and 6 swabs
   (C) 4 bandages and 5 swabs
   (D) 10 bandages and 8 swabs

4. A hospital maintenance department is installing new sanitary molding at the junction of the floor and the wall along both sides of a hallway. The plan drawing for the hallway has a scale of $\frac{1}{4}$ inch :1 foot. The hallway measures $7\frac{3}{4}$ inches long on the plan.

   How many pieces of 8-foot-long molding should the maintenance department order?

   (A) 4
   (B) 6
   (C) 7
   (D) 8

5. A medication is being administered to a client intravenously via a solution that has a 5% concentration of medication by volume of solution. At 8:00 AM, Alicia checked the remaining contents of the client's IV drip bag and noted that there were 780 cc of solution remaining. When she returned at 10:00 AM, there were 300 cc of the solution left in the IV bag. Which of the following correctly expresses the unit rate at which the medication is being dispensed?

   (A) $\dfrac{240 \text{ cc}}{\text{hour}}$

   (B) $\dfrac{24 \text{ cc}}{2 \text{ hours}}$

   (C) $\dfrac{2 \text{ cc}}{\text{minute}}$

   (D) $\dfrac{0.2 \text{ cc}}{\text{minute}}$

Review your work using the explanations in Part Six of this book.

LESSON 5

Estimating and Rounding

LEARNING OBJECTIVES

- Convert measurements between various metric units
- Round given quantities to a specified degree of precision
- Determine when estimating is an appropriate problem-solving strategy
- Use estimating to efficiently solve problems

Metric Units

The metric system of measurements has been widely adopted in medicine. The base units of measurement in the metric system are **meter** for length and **gram** for weight. A meter is about 10% longer than a yard, and a paper clip weighs about 1 gram. To have units that are appropriate to what is being measured, prefixes are used that correspond to the base unit times various powers of 10, as shown in this table:

Prefix	Power of 10	Unit Value
mega	10^6	1,000,000
kilo	10^3	1000
hecto	10^2	100
deca	10^1	10
deci	10^{-1}	0.1 or $\dfrac{1}{10}$
centi	10^{-2}	0.01 or $\dfrac{1}{100}$
milli	10^{-3}	0.001 or $\dfrac{1}{1000}$
micro	10^{-6}	0.000001 or $\dfrac{1}{1,000,000}$

By using a prefix, you can specify the exact unit of measurement. Because the different metric units are related by multiples of 10, converting from one unit to another is merely a matter of moving the decimal point and, if necessary, adding zeroes. For instance, to convert 1.75 kilograms to grams, multiply by 1000, which is $10 \times 10 \times 10$.

1.75 kilograms × 10 = 17.5 hectograms

17.5 hectograms × 10 = 175 decagrams

175 decagrams × 10 = 1750 grams

Similarly, to convert 23 millimeters to meters, multiply by 10^{-3}, an operation that is the same as dividing by 10 three times.

23 millimeters $\div$ 10 = 2.3 centimeters

2.3 centimeters $\div$ 10 = 0.23 decimeters

0.23 decimeters $\div$ 10 = 0.023 meters

Remember, when converting from larger units to smaller, there will be more of the smaller units, so you multiply; when converting from smaller units to larger ones, divide.

Metric area and volume measurements use the same units as length. Becuase area is, in its simplest terms, length times width, areas are expressed in units such as square meters (m^2). Similarly, volume is described in cubic units. A common such unit is cubic centimeters (abbreviated as cm^3 or cc). One measure of volume that is frequently used is the **liter**, which is 1000 cubic centimeters.

Rounding

Some questions on the TEAS will specifically direct you to round a given quantity or the results of calculations to a certain degree of accuracy. The rule for **rounding** is straightforward: if the digit following the one being rounded is 5 or greater, change it to 0 and add 1 to the previous digit. If the digit is less than 5, merely round down to 0. For example, to round 75 to the nearest multiple of 10 (the tens place; see Lesson 1: Arithmetic for a review), change the 5 to 0 and add 1 to the previous digit, 7, to obtain 80. To round 166.3 to the nearest whole number, just roll the 3 down to 0 to get 166.0, which is 166 to the nearest whole number.

When rounding by more than one digit, consider the whole amount that is being rounded. If you are rounding 847 to the nearest hundred, do not round the 7 up to get 850 and then round that up to 900. The digit actually being rounded is 4, so round down to 800.

Occasionally, rounding can involve quantities that are not decimal based. Pay close attention to the units involved. A common example is time. To round 3 hours 41 minutes to the nearest hour, don't just round down to 3 hours because 41 is less than 50. Instead, recall that an hour is 60 minutes so the quantity you are rounding is actually $3\frac{41}{60}$; because 41 is more than half of 60, round up to 4 hours.

This is the same technique that is used for rounding fractions. If the numerator is less than half the denominator, round down. If the numerator is greater than or equal to half the denominator, round up. For example, rounded to the nearest whole number, $3\frac{19}{32} \approx 4$ because 19 is greater than half of 32, but $3\frac{19}{46} \approx 3$ because 19 is less than half of 46.

Estimating

Estimating is a way to obtain approximate values for expressions by using rounding or other techniques to simplify the calculations. It is not guessing! The judicious use of estimating can save time and reduce errors. Rounding is a technique frequently used in estimating. If, for instance, a question required you to calculate the value of 37×53, you could estimate by rounding 37 to 40 and 53 to 50. Multiplying 40 times 50 gets 2000, very close to the actual value of 1961.

There are a few clues that you can use to decide whether estimating is an appropriate strategy. If you encounter a question with rather complex calculations that might be a candidate for estimating, take a glance at the answer choices to see if they are spaced far apart. For instance, if the choices for the above multiplication were 1224, 1611, 1961, 2335, and 2711, you could readily determine that 1961 was correct based on the estimated result of 2000. If, however, the choices were 1855, 1922, 1961, 2013, and 2131, merely estimating would not result in a correct answer. The question itself may also suggest when estimating is a good strategy. Wording such as "approximately," "closest to," or "about" might be a clue that you can arrive at the correct answer using estimating.

Study how an expert would apply these concepts to a test question.

Question	Analysis
Crystal has several pieces of pipe. She has 3 pieces that are 2.1 meters long, 5 that are 2.9 meters long, and 6 that are 4.1 meters long. How long would these pieces be if laid end to end?	**Step 1:** The question lists the lengths of several pieces of pipe and asks for their total length. A glance at the answer choices shows that they are spaced far enough apart that you can estimate the answer.
(A) 41.2 meters (B) 45.3 meters (C) 48.2 meters (D) 50.3 meters	**Step 2:** Round the lengths of the pipes. The total length will be about $(3 \times 2) + (5 \times 3) + (6 \times 4) = 6 + 15 + 24 = 45$ meters
	Step 3: The estimate of 45 meters is very close to the correct answer choice **(C)**, 45.3 meters.
	Step 4: Check your rounding and calculations and that you properly used the data in the question.

Be careful when using several rounded numbers to estimate, particularly in multiplication calculations. If a set of calculations required you to calculate $17 \times 8 \times 16$ and you estimated by rounding up all three numbers to 20, 10, and 20, your estimate would be 4000. However, the actual value is 2176. This big difference is due to the cumulative effect of multiplying three numbers that are all rounded up. However, if you used rounding to estimate 27×23 as $30 \times 20 = 600$, this would be a good approximation of the actual value, 621, because one number was rounded up and the other was rounded down.

Estimating can use techniques other than rounding. One such technique is to choose "compatible" numbers, that is, numbers that are easier to work with when calculating. For instance, to estimate $365 \div 73$, rather than just rounding to 370 and 70, use nearby compatible numbers of $350 \div 70$ to obtain an estimated value of 5.

Another technique that can be used either in combination with estimating or alone is rearranging. Look for opportunities to group sums into pairs that are easy to combine mentally. The most helpful rearrangements give you zeroes (through addition or subtraction) or multiples of 10.

Here's how an experienced test taker would use rearranging to simplify answering a question.

K

Question	Analysis
What is the value of $67 + 79 + 33$?	**Step 1:** The question adds three 2-digit numbers.
(A) 169 (B) 170 (C) 178 (D) 179	**Step 2:** You are asked to find the sum of those numbers. Before you begin adding, see whether any pairs of numbers might be added to get a nice round number; 67 and 33 end with digits that add up to 10. Indeed, 67 and 33 sum to 100. Now you can add the remaining number more easily: $100 + 79 = 179$.
	Step 3: Choice **(D)** matches.
	Step 4: Double-check the $67 + 33$ calculation to be certain that your tens digit is correct.

Rearranging requires a bit of extra thought up front, but you will increase your speed overall and reduce the chance of making a mistake. Avoid rearranging numbers in expressions that involve a combination of different operations and always follow PEMDAS.

Now you try an estimating question:

> Paula's car is low on gasoline, so she stops at a convenience store on her way home to buy gas and a few other items. She purchases a bottle of water for $1.69, 3 candy bars at 60¢ each, a sandwich for $2.29, and tissue for $2.69. Gasoline costs $2.49 per gallon. Paula only has $20 to spend. This particular store dispenses gasoline only by the gallon. How much gas can she add to her tank?
>
> (A) 3 gallons
> (B) 4 gallons
> (C) 5 gallons
> (D) 6 gallons

Explanation

Step 1: The question provides the prices of a few items and how much money is available to spend and asks how much will be left over to purchase gasoline. The answer will be stated to the nearest gallon, and the price per gallon is given.

Step 2: Due to the number of calculations required and the fact that the answer will be "to the nearest gallon," estimating is a good strategy. Rounding the prices, Paula will spend $1.70 + (3 \times 0.60) + 2.30 + 2.70$. Use PEMDAS and rearrange to get $1.70 + 2.30 + 1.80 + 2.70 = 4 + 4.50 = \$8.50$. Therefore, Paula will have about $11.50 left over to buy gasoline at about $2.50 per gallon. Try 5 gallons as a possible answer: $5 \times (2 + 0.50) = 10 + 2.50 = \$12.50$. Now try 4 gallons: $4 \times (2 + 0.50) = 8 + 2 = \$10.00$.

Step 3: Even though the $11.50 that Paula has available to buy gas is closer to the price of 5 gallons than to the amount needed to buy 4 gallons, the pump only dispenses by the gallon, so the most Paula could buy is **(B)**, 4 gallons. Choice (C) is a trap answer that ignores this detail.

Step 4: Double-check your logic, rounding, and calculations.

KEY IDEAS

- The metric system is decimal based, thus facilitating easy conversion between units.
- Rounding follows straightforward rules and can simplify calculations.
- Techniques that help solve problems include estimating, using compatible numbers, and rearranging.

Estimating and Rounding Practice Questions

1. What is the volume of 2753 cubic centimeters to the nearest liter?

   (A) 2
   (B) 3
   (C) 27
   (D) 28

2. What is the value of $(61 - 40) \times (36 - 18)$?

   (A) 189
   (B) 378
   (C) 641
   (D) 738

3. A leaky faucet drips water at a rate of 22 mL/hr. How much water drips from this faucet in 2 days?

   (A) 528 mL
   (B) 792 mL
   (C) 1056 mL
   (D) 1326 mL

4. There are 30 chocolate chip cookies in each package. A case consists of 24 packages. If the average breakage rate for these cookies is 1.72%, what would be the expected number of broken cookies per case, expressed as the nearest whole number?

   (A) 6
   (B) 10
   (C) 12
   (D) 15

5. What is the value of 27×43?

   (A) 1161
   (B) 1172
   (C) 1183
   (D) 1194

Review your work using the explanations in Part Six of this book.

Review and Reflect

Think about the questions you answered in these lessons.

- Were you able to approach each question systematically, using the Kaplan Method for Mathematics?
- Did you feel confident that you understood what the question was asking you to do?
- How well were you able to apply arithmetic and algebra rules to solving problems?
- Were there times when you could have solved more efficiently using critical thinking and estimation, rather than calculation?
- Did you confirm your answer for every question, checking that it made sense and that you had not made any arithmetic or algebra errors?
- If you missed any questions, do you understand why you got the incorrect answer? Could you do the question again now and get it right?

Use your thoughts about these questions to guide how you continue to prepare for the TEAS. If you feel you need more review and practice with arithmetic and algebra, you should study this chapter some more and use the online Qbank that comes with this book. After you have registered your book at **kaptest.com/booksonline**, log in to your student home page at **kaptest.com** to use your Qbank.

The TEAS also tests one other area of *Mathematics*:

- Statistics, Geometry, and Measurements

A chapter with lessons addressing these concepts and skills will be included in Kaplan's *ATI TEAS® Strategies, Practice, & Review with 2 Practice Tests*, which will be available for purchase in January 2017.

Science

Nursing and health science program professionals need to understand and be able to use knowledge about the human body as well as other scientific subjects. In your career, you will apply scientific knowledge frequently, and you will need to keep up-to-date on the latest published research to provide your clients with the best possible care. The TEAS *Science* content area tests your understanding of the parts and function of each organ system of the human body, and it asks questions about biology and chemistry. The TEAS also tests your ability to use scientific measurements and tools and to evaluate scientific research.

Questions by Content Area

Pie chart: English and language usage 17%, Reading 31%, Mathematics 21%, Science 31%

The TEAS Science Content Area

Of the 170 items on the TEAS, 53 will be in the *Science* content area, and you will have 63 minutes to answer them. Thus, you will have just over a minute (63 minutes ÷ 53 questions ≈ 1 minute 10 seconds) per question.

Of the 53 *Science* questions, 47 will be scored and 6 will be unscored. You won't know which questions are unscored, so do your best on every question.

The 47 scored *Science* questions come from three sub-content areas:

Sub-content areas	# of Questions
Human anatomy and physiology	32
Life and physical sciences	8
Scientific reasoning	7

Kaplan's *High-Yield Practice for the New ATI TEAS*® includes four lessons addressing areas of *Science* that the TEAS emphasizes:

- Chapter 1: Human Anatomy and Physiology
  - Lesson 1: Human Anatomy and Physiology: An Overview
  - Lesson 2: The Skeletal System
  - Lesson 3: The Neuromuscular System
  - Lesson 4: The Cardiovascular System

The Kaplan Method for Science

Using a methodical approach to *Science* questions will help you organize the relevant facts and eliminate incorrect answers.

> **Step 1:** Analyze the information provided.
>
> **Step 2:** Recall the relevant facts.
>
> **Step 3:** Predict the answer.
>
> **Step 4:** Evaluate the answer choices.

Step 1: Analyze the information provided.

Many questions on the TEAS ask you to recall science facts. In these cases, key terms are provided that tell you what area of science you are being tested on and which fact(s) you need to supply. If you are being asked to evaluate an experiment or draw a conclusion based on data or an experimental process, the data will be provided or the process described. This information, which may be in the question itself or in a table, figure, or other information supplied above the question, will be key to answering correctly, so invest enough time to study it carefully. In all cases, a glance at the answer choices may also provide useful guidance about the area of science being tested or the specificity of the answer sought.

Step 2: Recall the relevant facts.

The TEAS tests many topics in science. Therefore, each time you start a new question, give yourself the time it takes to orient yourself to the question's particular focus. Is it about the endocrine system? Heredity? The experimental method? Call to mind what you know about the topic.

If additional information is provided in the question or above it, then research it. It will either provide the answer to the question or facts you can use to deduce the answer. Read carefully! It would be a shame to know the material but miss the question because you, for example, misread the axis of a graph or named the independent variable instead of the dependent variable.

Step 3: Predict the answer.

By having the correct answer firmly in mind before you look at the answer choices, you will not choose an incorrect answer that looks similar or one that is a related concept but not the exact concept you need. Sometimes you may not know the science fact the question is asking for. Even in these cases, you can mentally review what you do remember about the topic. This will prepare you to eliminate clear wrong answers and increase your chance of getting the question right.

Step 4: Evaluate the answer choices.

Choose the answer choice that matches your prediction. If you were unable to make a prediction, eliminate those answer choices that relate to a different organ system or concept. This allows you to make a strategic guess among the remaining choices.

HUMAN ANATOMY AND PHYSIOLOGY

LEARNING OBJECTIVES

- Identify and describe the parts of the cell and the organization of the human body
- Identify features of the skeletal system, including types of bone and joints, and describe the structure and function of bone
- Identify the components of the neuromuscular system and describe their function, including muscular contraction
- Identify the parts of the cardiovascular system, describe their function, and trace the flow of blood in the body

Of the 47 scored *Science* questions, 32 (68%) will be in the sub-content area of *Human anatomy and physiology*. The TEAS tests your comprehension of the parts and function of human organ systems and your ability to apply this knowledge.

This chapter of *High-Yield Practice for the New ATI TEAS®* includes four lessons to address these topics:

Lesson 1: Human Anatomy and Physiology: An Overview

Lesson 2: The Skeletal System

Lesson 3: The Neuromuscular System

Lesson 4: The Cardiovascular System

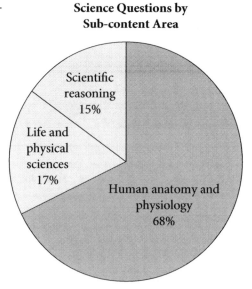

Science Questions by Sub-content Area

Scientific reasoning 15%

Life and physical sciences 17%

Human anatomy and physiology 68%

LESSON 1

Human Anatomy and Physiology: An Overview

LEARNING OBJECTIVES

- Identify and describe the functions of different cell parts
- Describe the organization of the body into tissues, organs, and organ systems
- Recognize anatomical positions, planes, and directions

Components of a Cell

Human cells are **eukaryotic**, meaning that they have a nucleus and membrane-bound **organelles** and are surrounded by a semipermeable **plasma membrane**. This membrane controls the movement of solutes into and out of the cell. The **nucleus** houses the cell's DNA and is surrounded by a double membrane. It is the site of DNA replication and RNA transcription. Outside the nucleus is the **cytoplasm**, an aqueous mixture of proteins and other biological molecules, which surrounds the other organelles. Each organelle has a specific cellular function, so the organelles can be thought of as miniature organs within the cell. The main organelles are summarized by function in the table.

Function	Organelle	Description
protein synthesis	**ribosomes**	Either free-floating in the cytoplasm or associated with the endoplasmic reticulum. They are composed of both ribosomal RNA and protein and translate messenger RNA into cellular proteins.
protein translation	**rough ER**	Contiguous with the nuclear membrane. It is studded with ribosomes and is the site of translation for membrane-bound or secreted proteins. Rough ER is also the site of protein folding and modification.
protein sorting and modification	**Golgi apparatus**	The site of sorting and packaging of proteins. This can be thought of as the cell's "post office." Proteins also undergo posttranslational modification as they transit through the Golgi apparatus.
ribosome assembly	**nucleolus**	Substructure of the nucleus. The nucleolus transcribes ribosomal RNA and combines ribosomal proteins to create the large and small ribosomal subunits.
waste breakdown	**lysosome**	Acidic compartments that contain hydrolytic enzymes and responsible for breaking down cellular waste. Lysosomes also play a role in the cellular defense against pathogens and apoptosis.

Function	Organelle	Description
energy production	**mitochondria**	Main powerhouse of the cell, producing ATP through aerobic respiration. Mitochondria have a double membrane, a small circular genome, and their own ribosomes.
cell organization	**centrosome**	Organizes the microtubules of the cell. The centrioles, a substructure in the centrosome, assemble the mitotic spindle during cell division.
detoxification and lipid synthesis	**smooth ER**	The smooth ER is contiguous with the nuclear membrane and produces lipids, phospholipids, and steroids. It also detoxifies metabolic by-products as well as alcohol and drugs. In muscle cells, it functions as a storage site for calcium.
locomotion	**cilia**	Celia are cellular protrusions that can beat to enable movement or serve to increase cell surface area to maximize absorption.

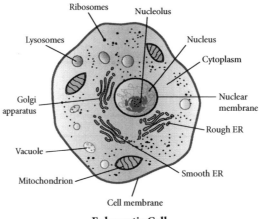

Eukaryotic Cell

Different cell types have different organelle compositions to better suit their individual functions. For example, muscle cells that require calcium for contraction have larger amounts of specialized smooth ER, which stores and releases calcium; they also have increased numbers of mitochondria to produce the ATP needed to sustain muscle contraction. Red blood cells lack all membrane-bound organelles so that they can hold large amounts of the oxygen-carrying protein hemoglobin.

Here is how an expert would answer a question about the organelles.

Question	Analysis
An inhibitor targeting the electron transport chain involved in ATP production would most likely target which organelle?	**Step 1:** This question is asking about the specific functions of the organelles. While you may not know specifically what the electron transport system is, the question stem states that it is involved in ATP production.
	Steps 2 and 3: Recall that the mitochondria of cells are responsible for ATP production. Predict mitochondria.
(A) Ribosomes	**Step 4:** Ribosomes are responsible for protein production. Eliminate.
(B) Golgi apparatus	The Golgi apparatus is responsible for protein modification and packaging. Eliminate.
(C) Mitochondria	Correct. The mitochondria are the main powerhouses of the cell and produce ATP.
(D) Centrosomes	The centrosomes are responsible for microtubule organization. Eliminate.

Tissues

Cells working together to perform a specific function form a **tissue**. There are four main tissue types found in the body.

Tissue Type	Description
epithelial	Epithelium serves two functions. It can provide covering (such as skin tissue) or produce secretions (such as glandular tissue). Epithelial tissue commonly exists in sheets and does not have its own blood supply. Subsequently, epithelium is dependent on diffusion from nearby capillaries for food and oxygen.
connective	Connective tissue is found throughout the body; it serves to connect and support different structures of the body. Connective tissue commonly has its own blood supply. The various types of connective tissue include bone, cartilage, adipose (fat), and blood vessel.
muscular	Muscle tissue is dedicated to producing movement. There are three types of muscle tissue: skeletal, cardiac, and smooth.
nervous	Nervous tissue provides the structure for the brain, spinal cord, and nerves. Nerves are made up of specialized cells called neurons that send electrical impulses throughout the body.

Organs and Organ Systems

An **organ** is a structure composed of multiple tissue types working together to perform a specific function; for example, the lungs oxygenate blood, and the kidneys filter blood. Organs can be further grouped together into **organ systems**, in which multiple organs work together to perform a larger function. There are 10 main organ systems in the body: respiratory, digestive, immune, endocrine, circulatory, urinary, reproductive, muscular, nervous, and skeletal systems. A summary of their function is provided in the table.

Organ System	Components	Function
respiratory	nose, throat, and lungs	Takes in oxygen and releases carbon dioxide.
digestive	mouth, esophagus, stomach, small and large intestine	Breaks down foods into nutrients that can be absorbed.
immune	spleen, bone marrow, lymph nodes	Protects the body from foreign pathogens.
endocrine	hypothalamus, pituitary, adrenal glands, thyroid, testes, ovaries, pancreas	Produces and secretes hormones to control bodily processes, including glucose regulation, sleep cycles, and gametogenesis.
urinary	kidneys, ureters, bladder, urethra	Filters blood and eliminates waste through urine.
reproductive	Males: testes, penis Females: ovaries, uterus, vagina	Produces gametes and facilitates fertilization.
muscular	muscle	Enables movement of the body.
nervous	brain, spinal cord, nerves	Receives and processes stimuli, transmits information, controls bodily functions.
skeletal	bones	Protects internal organs, creates blood cells, provides a framework for muscle.
circulatory	heart and blood vessels	Moves blood throughout the body to enable nutrient delivery to and waste removal from tissues.

Anatomical Planes and Terminology

Anatomical planes divide the body into distinct halves. Resting pose is defined as a human standing with feet parallel and facing forward, with arms at sides, palms facing forward and fingers pointing down. There are three main anatomic planes.

Plane	Description
coronal plane	Runs vertically and separates the body into front and back halves.
sagittal plane	Runs vertically and separates the body into left and right halves. Note that the left-right division is in relation to the body, not the view looking at the body from the front. In other words, your right hand is on the right side of your body.
transverse plane	Runs horizontally and divides the body into top and bottom halves; also called the *axial plane* or *horizontal plane*.

Directional terminology is used to describe the locations of different parts of the human body. Common terms include those in the table.

Term	Definition	Example
superior	The top half of the body along the transverse plane	The head is on the superior axis.
inferior	The bottom half of the body along the transverse plane	The foot is on the inferior axis.
anterior/ventral	The front part of the body along the coronal plane	The clavicle is on the ventral side of the body.
posterior/dorsal	The back part of the body along the coronal plane	The shoulder blades are on the posterior side of the body.
medial	Toward the midline of the body along the sagittal plane	The thumb is on the lateral side of the body.
lateral	Away from the midline of the body along the sagittal plane	The pinky finger is on the medial side of the body.
proximal	Toward the post of origin	The proximal convoluted tubule is closest to the Bowman's capsule.
distal	Away from the point of origin	The distal convoluted tubule is farthest away from the Bowman's capsule.

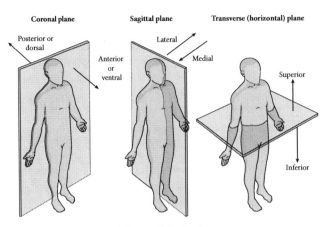

Planes of the Body

Directional terms can also be combined to better describe the location of a body part. For example, the nose is both ventral and superior.

Now you try this question on directional terminology.

The collar bone is located on the _____ side of the body.

(A) superior and dorsal
(B) superior and ventral
(C) inferior and dorsal
(D) inferior and ventral

Explanation

Step 1: This question is asking about the location of the collar bone. Based on the answer options, you need to determine its place relative to the coronal and transverse planes.

Step 2: Recall that the coronal plane divides the body into dorsal and ventral halves and the transverse plane divides the body into superior and inferior halves.

Step 3: The collar bone is on the ventral side of the coronal plane and the superior side of the transverse plane.

Step 4: Answer choice **(B)** matches this prediction.

KEY IDEAS

- Eukaryotic cells contain membrane-bound organelles, and each organelle performs a specific function or set of functions in the cell.
- Cells are organized into tissues that serve a specific task. Tissues working together for a common function comprise organs. Organ systems are the highest level of organization within the body and are comprised of multiple organs that perform different tasks.
- The body can be subdivided along multiple planes, and specific directional terms can be used to describe the location of different body parts.

Human Anatomy and Physiology: An Overview Practice Questions

1. A macrophage, a type of immune cell responsible for phagocytosing and digesting pathogens, is likely to contain more of which of the following organelles?

    (A) Mitochondria
    (B) Lysosomes
    (C) Ribosomes
    (D) Centrosomes

2. A buildup of urea, a nitrogenous waste product of protein metabolism, in the body is most likely due to the failure of which organ system?

    (A) Urinary
    (B) Endocrine
    (C) Digestive
    (D) Immune

3. The _____ plane runs horizontally through the body and divides it into inferior and superior halves.

    (A) medial
    (B) coronal
    (C) sagittal
    (D) transverse

Review your work using the explanations in Part Six of this book.

LESSON 2

The Skeletal System

LEARNING OBJECTIVES

- Identify specific structures of the skeletal system
- Explain how the muscular system works with the skeletal system to move the body
- Classify different types of joints
- Describe the microscopic and macroscopic structure of bone

The skeletal system has multiple functions in the body including protecting internal organs, facilitating movement, creating new blood cells, and metabolism.

Parts of the Skeleton

The skeletal system can be broken down into two main divisions: axial and appendicular. The **axial skeleton** consists of the skull, vertebrae, rib cage, and hyoid bone and provides the general scaffold of the body. The **appendicular skeleton** consists of the limb bones, scapula, clavicle, and pelvis and enables movement. The names of the specific bones of the body, as well as their location, are shown here. The TEAS may provide you with a diagram and expect you to be able to identify these bones.

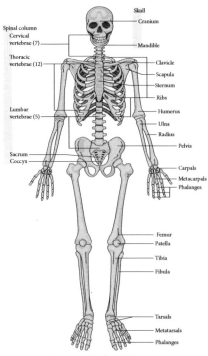

Human Skeletal System

There are four main types of bone: long, short, flat, and irregular.

- **Long bones** are hollow, filled with marrow, and longer than they are wide. They function to support the weight of the body and facilitate movement. They are largely part of the appendicular skeleton and include the femur, tibia, fibula, metatarsals, phalanges, humerus, radius, and metacarpals.
- **Short bones** are wider than they are long and provide stability and some movement. They include the carpals and tarsals.
- **Flat bones** provide protection to internal organs and function as areas of attachment for muscles. They include the sternum, ribs, and pelvis.
- **Irregular bones** vary in their structure and shape and thus do not fit into any other category. They include the bones of the vertebral column, the skull, and the knee and elbow.

Bones are connected at joints via **ligaments**. The hyoid bone, which supports the tongue, is the only bone in the body supported solely by muscle. The articulating ends of bone, or points of contact, are covered with **hyaline cartilage** to prevent direct bone contact and cushion the joint. There are three main types of joints:

- **Synovial joints**, including the ball-and-socket, hinge, and pivot joints, are the most common joint in the body and contain lubricating **synovial fluid**. Types of synovial joints include the knee, elbow, hip, and shoulder joints.
- **Fibrous joints** are held together only by ligaments and are not movable. Examples are the joints of the bones in the skull.
- **Cartilaginous joints** occur when two bones meet at a connection made of cartilage and are partially movable, such as joints between vertebrae in the spine.

Arthritis develops when cartilage between joints breaks down over time or as the result of joint inflammation. **Rheumatoid arthritis**, an autoimmune disease, is caused by immune cells attacking either the cartilage or joint lining, leading to bone erosion and pain.

Here is how an expert would answer a question about the skeletal system.

Question	Analysis
Which of the following is NOT classified as a synovial joint?	**Step 1:** This question is asking which is *not* synovial, so three answer choices will be synovial, and the correct answer choice will not be.
	Step 2: Recall that synovial joints are movable joints. Types of synovial joints are the pivot, the ball-and-socket, and the hinge.
	Step 3: Eliminate answers that fall into these categories.
(A) Femur and pelvis	**Step 4:** The femur and pelvis meet at a ball-and-socket joint. Eliminate
(B) Skull bones	Correct. The skull bones are not movable and join at fibrous, not synovial joints.
(C) Humerus and ulna	The humerus and ulna meet at a hinge joint. Eliminate.
(D) Humerus and scapula	The humerus and scapula meet at a ball-and-socket joint. Eliminate.

The skeletal system also provides a structural framework onto which muscles can attach to move the body. Muscles attach to bone via **tendons.** Tendons are the fibrous connective tissue that attach muscle to bone. At least two muscles attach at the joint of each movable limb and move the limb through antagonistic contraction, in which one muscle contracts and the antagonistic muscle relaxes. The bicep and tricep, for example, are antagonistic muscles. To move the forearm closer to the body, the bicep contracts and the tricep relaxes, but to extend the forearm away from the body, the bicep relaxes and the tricep contracts.

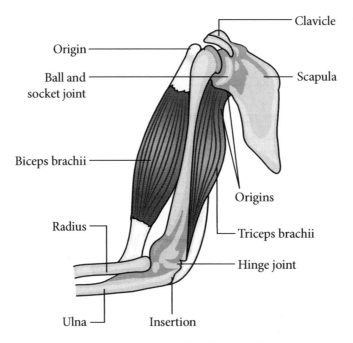

Antagonistic Muscle Pair: The Biceps and Triceps

Macroscopic Structure of Bone

There are two main types of bone tissue: spongy and compact. **Spongy bone,** which is less dense than compact bone and is located in the ends of bones, contains **bone marrow,** the site of red blood cell (erythrocyte) and lymphocyte production. **Compact bone** is much denser; it supports the body and stores calcium.

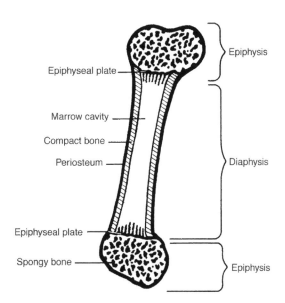

Basic Structure of Bone

Long bones are characterized by a cylindrical shaft, called the **diaphysis**, and dilated ends, called the **epiphyses**. The diaphysis is mainly composed of compact bone, which surrounds a hollow cavity containing the bone marrow. The epiphyses are composed of spongy bone surrounding a layer of compact bone. The **epiphyseal plate**, the growth plate, is the site of new bone growth. The **periosteum**, a fibrous sheath, surrounds and protects the bone.

Now you try this question about the skeletal system.

A defect in which of the following parts of bone would be most likely to result in stunted growth?

(A) Diaphysis
(B) Epiphysis
(C) Epiphyseal plate
(D) Periosteum

Explanation

Step 1: This question is testing your knowledge of the different bone components, specifically the site where bone growth occurs.

Step 2: Recall that new bone is made at the epiphyseal plate, or growth plate. A defect in new bone growth would cause stunted growth.

Step 3: Predict epiphyseal plate.

Step 4: Select answer choice **(C).**

Microscopic Structure of Bone

Bone is much more dynamic than you might think—approximately 10 percent of the human skeleton is replaced each year through the action of osteoblasts and osteoclasts. **Osteoblasts** build bone, while **osteoclasts** break it down. A great mnemonic is that *blasts build and clasts cleave*. **Osteocytes**, another type of bone cell, are responsible for sensing mechanical stress and regulate both osteoblasts and osteoclasts.

Bone is a vascularized, mineralized matrix containing a calcium phosphate collagen matrix. Bone is synthesized as **osteons**, cylindrical structures comprised of concentric rings of a mineralized matrix known as **lamellae**. **Haversian canals** run down the center of each osteon and contain blood vessels that provide nutrients to the bone cells (the osteoblasts, osteoclasts, and osteocytes). **Volkmann canals** connect the Haversian canals, enabling nutrient exchange between osteons. Cells reside in **lacunae**, spaces found between the lamellae. Microscopic channels, **canaliculi**, connect the lacunae to enable cellular communication.

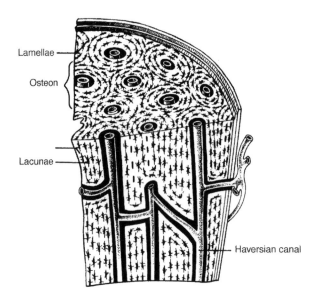

Diseases of the bone include the following:

- **Osteoporosis**, a loss in bone mineral density, is caused by lack of calcium and vitamin D in the body, as well as bone loss that occurs naturally with aging.
- **Osteogenesis imperfecta**, also known as brittle bone disease, is a genetic disease whereby either insufficient or defective collagen is produced, making bones very fragile and easy to break.
- **Osteoarthritis** is a degenerative joint disease characterized by the loss of cushioning cartilage.

Now try this question on the skeletal system.

An overactivation of which of the following bone cells could lead to osteoporosis?

(A) Osteon
(B) Osteoblast
(C) Osteoclast
(D) Osteocyte

Explanation

Step 1: The answer choices for this question are all different bone cells, and you are asked which one would most likely contribute to a disease of bone.

Step 2: Recall that osteoporosis results from a demineralization of bone. Thus, the function of the cell responsible for osteoporosis must be breaking down bone.

Step 3: Predict that osteoclasts "cleave" or break down bone.

Step 4: Select answer choice **(C).**

KEY IDEAS

- The skeleton can be subdivided into axial and appendicular, and it is comprised of four main types of bone: long, short, flat, and irregular.
- The most common type of joint in the body is the synovial joint; examples are ball-and-socket, hinge, and pivot joints.
- Compact bone is dense and supports the body, while spongy bone contains bone marrow, where certain blood cells are made.
- Bone is a highly dynamic tissue, as it is broken down by osteoclasts and built by osteoblasts.

Skeletal System Practice Questions

1. Drugs designed to treat osteoporosis would most likely increase the activity of which of the following bone cells?

   (A) Osteoblast
   (B) Osteoclast
   (C) Osteocyte
   (D) Osteon

2. Which of the following bones can be characterized as a long bone?

   (A) Carpal
   (B) Humerus
   (C) Pelvis
   (D) Vertebra

Review your work using the explanations in Part Six of this book.

LESSON 3

The Neuromuscular System

LEARNING OBJECTIVES

- Identify the components of the neuromuscular system and state their role(s)
- Differentiate between the central nervous system and the peripheral nervous system
- Describe the sequence of events that occur before, during, and after muscle contraction

The neuromuscular system consists of the nervous system and muscular system. Working together, these two systems are responsible for coordinating every movement of the body.

Anatomy of the Nervous System

The **nervous system** allows the body to sense and respond to environmental changes, both those that arise internally as well as those caused by external stimuli. This system consists of two parts: the central nervous system, comprised of the brain and spinal cord, and the peripheral nervous system, consisting of **neurons** (nerve cells) that send and receive signals throughout the body.

The **central nervous system** (CNS) processes information in the brain. The brain functions as the control center for the body and occupies the cranium, or skull.

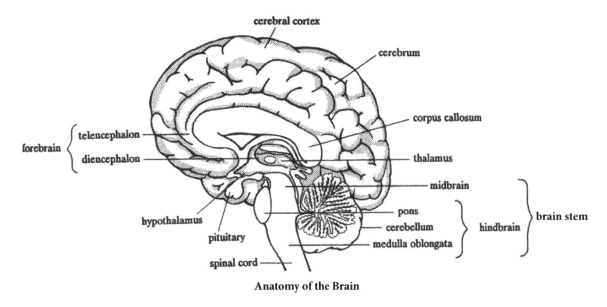

Anatomy of the Brain

The largest part of the brain is the **cerebrum**, which is responsible for thought and perception as well as visual and auditory processing. The cerebrum is divided into two halves, connected by nerve fibers that form the **corpus callosum**, which are further subdivided into four lobes: frontal, parietal, occipital, and temporal.

The **brain stem** connects the cerebrum to the spinal cord and controls critical involuntary body functions. Muscle control and balance are coordinated by the **cerebellum**, a dense cluster of neurons located at the base of the brain. The **medulla** regulates breathing, swallowing, and the beating of the heart.

Nerve impulses are transmitted from the extremities of the body to the brain via the **spinal cord**, a cylindrical column of nerves that runs through the center of the spine. **Spinal nerves** contain both **sensory fibers** and **motor fibers**. Sensory information such as temperature, pain, or pressure is conveyed to the brain along **afferent (sensory) neurons**. Response commands from the CNS are transmitted back to the musculature along **efferent (motor) neurons**.

The **peripheral nervous system** includes all nerves that exist outside the CNS. It can be further divided into the **somatic nervous system**, which sends and receives signals from skeletal muscle, which is under conscious control, and the **autonomic nervous system**, which regulates body processes that do not require conscious control. These include smooth and cardiac muscle activity and glandular secretions. The **sympathetic** division of the autonomic nervous system controls the body's "fight or flight" response to threat. The **parasympathetic** division returns the body to its resting state. These two systems work in opposition to one another.

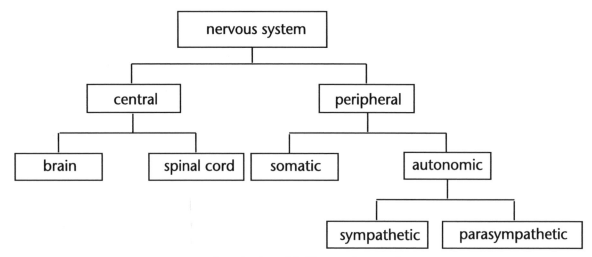

Organization of the Nervous System

There are 12 sets of **cranial nerves** that reach the interior of the brain, each with a specific function. For instance, the **optic nerve** transmits visual stimuli from your eye to your brain, allowing you to see, and the **vagus nerve** conveys signals from your abdominal organs, controlling digestion and heart rate among other parasympathetic responses. **Spinal nerves** transmit both sensory and motor signals from the spinal cord to a specific area of the body. The largest spinal nerve is the **sciatic nerve**, which runs from the lower spinal column down the leg. Peripheral nerve damage, or **neuropathy**, can lead to muscle weakness, tingling sensations, numbness, or paralysis depending on the degree and location of the injury.

Here is how an expert would answer a question about the nervous system.

Question	Analysis
The autonomic nervous system would be involved in all of the following EXCEPT	**Step 1:** This question is asking about specific actions of the autonomic nervous system.
	Step 2: Recall that the autonomic nervous system carries impulses between smooth and cardiac muscle and the central nervous system. Therefore, all actions involving smooth or cardiac muscle will be controlled by the autonomic nervous system.
	Step 3: Predict that the correct answer to this EXCEPT question will involve skeletal muscle.
(A) digesting a meal.	**Step 4:** Digestion is an involuntary process involving the smooth muscle of the stomach and intestines and glandular secretions of the pancreas and gallbladder. Eliminate.
(B) exhaling after holding your breath.	Breathing is regulated by the autonomic nervous system, even though temporary voluntary control—such as holding your breath—can be initiated. The smooth muscle of the lungs would be signaled to exhale if receptors recognized a buildup of CO_2 in the bloodstream.
(C) maintaining blood pressure.	Blood pressure is regulated by the involuntary contraction or dilation of blood vessels, under the control of the autonomic nervous system.
(D) jerking away from a painful stimulus.	Reacting to a painful stimulus is a reflex action under involuntary control. However, reflex actions are controlled by skeletal muscle. This is therefore *not* regulated by the autonomic nervous system. Choice **(D)** is correct.

Anatomy of the Muscular System

There are three types of muscle in the **muscular system**: skeletal, smooth, and cardiac. Each muscle is an organ containing muscle tissue, connective tissue, nervous tissue, and blood.

Skeletal muscle is composed of multiple **fascicles**, bundles of cells surrounded by connective tissue. Each fascicle contains multiple muscle fibers, or cells. These muscle fibers appear striated, or striped, due to the alignment of sarcomeres within each **myofibril**. **Sarcomeres**, which are the contractile unit of the muscle cell, are composed of **actin**, the thin filament protein, and **myosin**.

The largest skeletal muscle in the body is the **gluteus maximus**, which straightens the leg at the hip and helps keep the body upright. The smallest muscle is the the **stapedius**. This 1 mm long muscle stabilizes the bone in the middle ear and controls the conduction of sound waves into the inner ear.

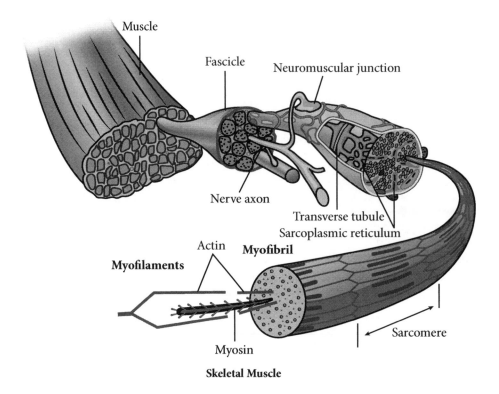

Muscle

Fascicle Neuromuscular junction

Nerve axon

Transverse tubule
Sarcoplasmic reticulum

Actin **Myofibril**

Myofilaments

Myosin

Skeletal Muscle

Smooth muscle lacks striations and is responsible for involuntary muscular contraction in the walls of hollow visceral organs, like the gastrointestinal tract, and in blood vessels. Actin and myosin are both present, but they are not organized into bundles of sarcomeres. Instead, they are arranged in a diagonal spiral, which causes the muscle to twist, rather than shorten, upon contraction.

Cardiac muscle occurs only in the heart. Like smooth muscle, cardiac muscle is also under involuntary contraction. Unlike smooth muscle, cardiac cells are striated and contain myofibrils and **T tubules**. Cardiac muscle is distinguishable from skeletal muscle because it consists of branching chains of striated cells and individual cardiac cells are not regulated by individual neuromuscular junctions.

If muscle is deprived of oxygen for an extended period of time, it will become **ischemic,** meaning the muscle tissue has become damaged or has died as a result of inadequate blood flow. In cardiac muscle, this event is often referred to as a heart attack.

Now try answering this question about the muscular system:

Which of the following neuromuscular processes are involved in chemical digestion?
(A)   Autonomic control by the sciatic nerve
(B)   Somatic control by the vagus nerve
(C)   Smooth muscle contraction in the small intestine
(D)   Skeletal muscle contraction in the stomach

Explanation

Step 1: This question is asking about the nerves and muscles that control chemical digestion.

Step 2: Recall that chemical digestion is an involuntary process that occurs primarily in the stomach and intestines.

Step 3: Predict that the correct answer will involve either smooth muscle or autonomic nerves.

Step 4: Only answer choice **(C)** matches your prediction. The sciatic nerve controls skeletal muscle. While the vagus nerve is involved in digestion, it is involved in the autonomic nervous system, not the somatic nervous system. The stomach is also comprised of smooth muscle.

Neural Regulation of Muscle Contraction

Each neuron has a cell body, called the **soma**, multiple branched **dendrites**, and an **axon**. Messages are communicated between the brain and the muscular system by way of electrical signals called **action potentials** that travel along the axon. The process of generating an action potential, called **polarization**, can be triggered when a dendrite receives an impulse from a sensory receptor. Action potentials occur in an "all or none" fashion. Either one is triggered or one isn't.

Most axons are insulated with layers of **myelin**, which helps to increase the speed of the electrical impulse along the nerve cell. Demyelinating disorders, such as multiple sclerosis, prevent these impulses from being transmitted effectively and can result in uncoordinated muscle movement.

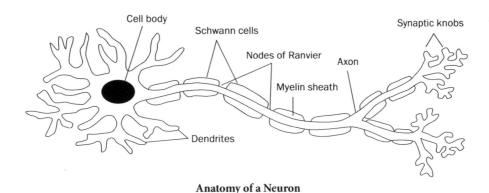

Anatomy of a Neuron

The space between the axon of one neuron and the dendrite of another is called the **synapse**. Neurons communicate across the synapse using **neurotransmitters**. At the synapse between a motor neuron and muscle fiber, or the **neuromuscular junction**, the specific neurotransmitter released is called **acetylcholine**, or ACh. In skeletal muscle, acetylcholine triggers the release of Ca^{2+}, which causes the actin and myosin to interact. A single motor neuron can communicate to numerous muscle fibers at once, defined as the **motor unit.**

During muscle **contraction**, the myosin head binds to actin, shortening the sarcomere as the thin filament is pulled over the thick filament. Like action potentials, muscle contraction is triggered in an "all or none" fashion. When contraction is signaled, all fibers of the motor unit contract at full force. The overall force of the muscular contraction varies by how many motor units are contracted simultaneously. Muscles that are not used regularly may **atrophy**; the myofibrils will shrink, resulting in weaker muscular contractions. After prolonged periods of disuse, the nerve supply to atrophied muscle tissue is reduced, and musculature is irreversibly replaced with connective tissue.

Muscle fatigue can result when a muscle is exerted strenuously over a long period. This can result from a depletion of ACh at the neuromuscular junction, meaning that contraction can no longer be signaled, or from a buildup of **lactic acid**, which impairs the muscle's ability to contract due to changes in muscle tissue pH. **Muscle strain** occurs when muscle fibers are overstretched or torn.

Now use what you know about muscle contraction to answer the following question:

Muscle contraction will occur only if

    (A)   acetylcholine is released by the dendrite.
    (B)   an action potential travels down the axon.
    (C)   all the motor units are activated.
    (D)   the muscle tissue is polarized.

Explanation

Step 1: This question is asking about the process of initiating muscle contraction.

Step 2: Recall that muscle contraction begins with the polarization of the dendrite and ends with the binding of actin and myosin.

Step 3: Predict that the answer will involve a true statement about the sequence of events in muscle contraction.

Step 4: Choice **(B)** matches your prediction. ACh is released at the synapse, not the dendrite, and is only one of many neurotransmitters. While motor units always contract in an all-or-none fashion, a muscle may contract when only some of its motor units are activated; if only a few units are activated, the contraction will be weak. It is the polarization of the neuron, not the muscle tissue, that initiates contraction.

KEY IDEAS

- Neurons coordinate all movements of the body by carrying messages between the nervous system and the muscular system.
- There are three types of muscle tissue. Skeletal muscle is under voluntary control. Smooth and cardiac muscle are under involuntary control.
- Muscle contraction occurs when an action potential in the neuron triggers the release of neurotransmitter at the synapse. This, in turn, leads to the binding of actin and myosin in the sarcomere.

Neuromuscular System Practice Questions

1. Signals from touch receptors in the hand are transmitted to the brain via

   (A) an afferent neuron.
   (B) the brain stem.
   (C) an efferent neuron.
   (D) a motor neuron.

2. Damage to the cerebellum would most likely result in

   (A) speech impairment.
   (B) difficulty walking.
   (C) loss of short-term memory.
   (D) life-threatening injury.

3. Which of these statements is correct regarding muscle contraction?

   (A) When a person is at rest, no muscles are contracting.
   (B) Muscle contraction is activated by actin and myelin cross-bridges.
   (C) Sensory neurons stimulate muscle tissue to contract.
   (D) Muscle fibers contract in an all-or-none fashion.

Review your work using the explanations in Part Six of this book.

LESSON 4

The Cardiovascular System

LEARNING OBJECTIVES

- Identify the components of the cardiovascular system and state their function(s)
- Trace the flow of blood through the cardiovascular system
- Describe how the cardiovascular system is regulated

The cardiovascular system supplies oxygen and nutrients to every living cell throughout the body by orchestrating movement of blood and lymph.

Anatomy of the Cardiovascular System

The cardiovascular system, also called the circulatory system, is composed of the heart, blood vessels, and blood.

The **heart** propels blood through the blood vessels and is the key organ of the circulatory system. There are four muscular chambers of the heart: the right and left atria and the right and left ventricles. The **atria** receive blood returning to the heart from other areas of the body, and the **ventricles** collect and expel blood from the heart. The atria and ventricles are separated by **atrioventricular valves**: the **tricuspid valve** separates the right atrium and right ventricle, and the **mitral valve** (also called **bicuspid**) separates the left atrium and left ventricle. As you learned in Lesson 3, the heart is composed of cardiac muscle tissue.

Blood outside the heart travels through the blood vessels. There are three major types of blood vessels: arteries, capillaries, and veins. **Arteries** are strong, elastic vessels adapted to the high pressure of blood as it leaves the heart. Smaller branches of the arteries (called **arterioles**) supply blood to the **capillaries**, the smallest blood vessels. Capillaries consist of only a single layer of epithelial tissue. This allows substances and gases to be exchanged between the blood and the cells of tissues via **diffusion**. The largest artery in the body is the **aorta**.

Blood returns to the heart from the capillaries via **venules**, which merge to form veins. The walls of **veins** are thinner than those of arteries because veins do not have to carry blood under high pressure. Veins also contain valves to prevent the backflow of blood. The largest vein in the body is the **inferior vena cava**, which brings deoxygenated blood back to the heart. The **pulmonary veins**, which bring blood from the lungs to the heart, are the among the few veins that carry oxygenated blood.

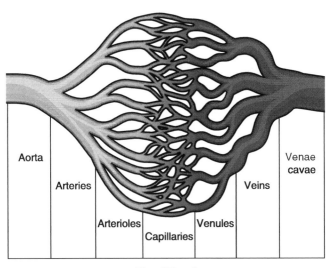

Blood Vessels

Blood is an essential bodily fluid that transports oxygen and nutrients to the tissues and removes waste products, including carbon dioxide and ammonia. There are four main components of human blood: red blood cells, white blood cells, platelets, and plasma.

All blood components are suspended in a matrix of **plasma,** the liquid component of blood that accounts for approximately half the blood volume. In addition to the blood cells, plasma contains proteins and electrolytes.

Red blood cells, or **erythrocytes,** account for the second greatest component of blood by volume. The functional unit of an erythrocyte is **hemoglobin,** an iron-containing protein that facilitates gas exchange by binding to oxygen or carbon dioxide. **Anemia** is a condition that occurs when hemoglobin levels are low, either because the body isn't producing enough red blood cells, such as when someone has iron deficiency, or because of another underlying condition that causes the red blood cells to be irregularly shaped, such as the **sickle-cell** trait.

White blood cells, called **leukocytes,** are part of the body's immune response and remove pathogens and foreign material from the blood. There are several different types of white blood cell, each with its own function. **Lymphocytes,** for example, release antibodies in response to disease and harness other immune system responses.

Platelets are cell fragments that prevent bleeding by developing blood clots. They work with coagulating proteins to stick to vessel walls and to each other. Having too few platelets, a condition called **thrombocytopenia,** can result in excessive external bleeding, such as nosebleeds, or in bruising caused by uncontrolled bleeding under the skin.

Here is how an expert would answer a question about the circulatory system.

Question	Analysis
Which of the following blood component levels would be expected to increase in response to a viral infection?	**Step 1:** This question is asking about the role of each blood component.
	Step 2: Recall that lymphocytes release antibodies as part of the immune response to disease or infection.

Question	Analysis
	Step 3: Predict the correct answer will correctly refer to the lymphocyte.
(A) Erythrocytes	**Step 4:** This is a red blood cell, the oxygen-transporting component of blood. Eliminate.
(B) Leukocytes	Correct. Leukocytes are white blood cells, of which lymphocytes are one specific type.
(C) Plasma	Plasma makes up the majority of the blood volume, which does not change as a result of infection. Eliminate.
(D) Platelets	Platelets are the blood-clotting component. Eliminate.

Paths of Circulation

The **closed circulatory system** is often described as a double loop because blood flows through the heart twice: once in its oxygenated state on its way to the body and once more when it is deoxygenated and on its way to the lungs. These two pathways are called the systemic circuit and the pulmonary circuit.

The **systemic circuit** carries oxygenated blood away from the left ventricle of the heart and returns deoxygenated blood to right atrium. The systemic circuit includes the aorta and blood vessels leading to the body tissues, as well as all the veins and venae cavae.

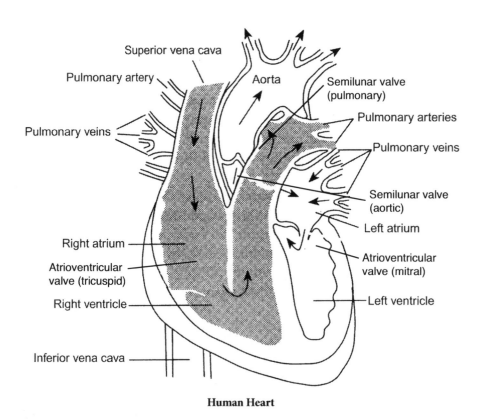

Human Heart

The **pulmonary circuit** contains the blood vessels that carry blood to and from the lungs. Deoxygenated blood flows from the right ventricle through the pulmonary arteries to the lungs, where the blood picks up oxygen. It then returns to the left atrium via the pulmonary vein.

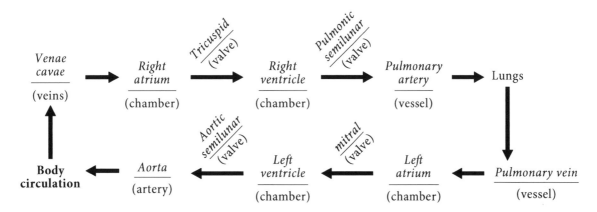

Double-Loop Circulation

The open circulatory system, or **lymphatic system**, is a network of capillaries that drain toxins and wastes away from the body tissues into the blood and plays a vital role in monitoring and removing foreign entities in the body. Waste products are absorbed into the **lymph**, a clear plasma-like fluid high in white blood cells, and filtered through one of several **lymph nodes**, which contain high concentrations of lymphocytes. The lymph is eventually drained into the subclavian veins.

Now you try answering a question on circulatory pathways.

> Which of the following statements regarding the pulmonary arteries is correct?
>
> (A) They carry oxygenated blood away from the heart.
> (B) They carry oxygenated blood away from the lungs.
> (C) They carry deoxygenated blood to the heart.
> (D) They carry deoxygenated blood to the lungs.

Explanation

Step 1: This question is asking about properties of the pulmonary arteries, specifically the direction of blood flow and the oxygenation status of the blood.

Step 2: Recall that arteries transport blood away from the heart. The pulmonary artery is transporting blood away from the heart to the lungs, so the blood is deoxygenated at this time.

Step 3: Predict that the correct answer will be away from the heart in an deoxygenated state.

Step 4: Your prediction matches answer **(D)**.

Cardiovascular Regulation

The **cardiac cycle** describes the period between the start of one heartbeat and the beginning of the next. Unlike skeletal muscle, cardiac muscle does not rely upon neural stimulation to initiate a contraction; cardiac muscle tissue can generate and conduct its own electrical impulses and can contract on its own.

There are two phases to the cardiac cycle: systole (contraction) and diastole (relaxation). During **systole**, contraction forces the blood to move from the chamber either into another heart chamber or into an artery. Atrial systole will move blood into the relaxed ventricles, whereas ventricular systole will pump blood into either the aorta or pulmonary artery, once the pressure of contraction opens the semilunar valves. During **diastole**, the heart muscle relaxes, and the chambers are passively filled with blood. The alternating closures of the atrioventricular and semilunar valve are responsible for the distinct "lub-dub" sound of the heartbeat. **Congestive heart failure** develops when the heart can no longer pump blood effectively, such as when weakened heart valves permit the backflow of blood into the chambers.

A reading of **blood pressure**, the pressure of the blood in the circulatory system, has two numbers (e.g., 120/80) to reflect the different pressures that occur at systole and diastole. Blood pressure is maintained by adjusting cardiac output and vascular resistance. If blood pressure begins to increase, the medulla will signal the heart to beat slower. Likewise, if blood pressure begins to drop, heart rate will increase to adjust.

Chronic high blood pressure, or **hypertension,** can result from multiple factors, including **atherosclerosis** (narrowing of the arteries due to plaque buildup), increased blood viscosity (such as if the blood contains high levels of cholesterol), and heart disease.

KEY IDEAS

- The heart regulates blood flow through a double-loop system, pumping oxygenated blood to the body tissue and deoxygenated blood to the lungs.
- Blood transports oxygen (via hemoglobin) and nutrients throughout the body by way of the circulatory system.
- Lymph, which moves through the open circulatory system before draining into the veins near the heart, contains infection-fighting white blood cells.

Cardiovascular System Practice Questions

1. Which of the following valves prevents blood from backflowing between the right atrium and right ventricle?

   (A) Aortic
   (B) Bicuspid
   (C) Mitral
   (D) Tricuspid

2. Which of the following correctly describes the flow of blood through the double-loop system?

   (A) Left ventricle - right ventricle - capillaries - pulmonary vein - right atrium
   (B) Left ventricle - pulmonary vein - lungs - pulmonary artery - right ventricle
   (C) Left ventricle - aorta - capillaries - vena cava - right ventricle
   (D) Left ventricle - arteries - veins - right ventricle - right atrium

3. Which of the following blood particles are responsible for blood clotting?

   (A) Platelets
   (B) Antibodies
   (C) Hemoglobin
   (D) Lymph

Review your work using the explanations in Part Six of this book.

Review and Reflect

Think about the questions you answered in these lessons.

- Were you able to approach each question systematically, using the Kaplan Method for Science?
- Did you feel confident that you understood what the question was asking you to do?
- Were you able to recall the facts the question was asking for?
- How well were you able to predict an answer before looking at the answer choices?
- Could you match your prediction to the correct answer?
- Are there areas of science that appear on the TEAS that you don't understand as well as you would like?
- If you missed any questions, do you understand why the answer you chose is incorrect and why the right answer is correct? Could you do the question again now and get it right?

Use your thoughts about these questions to guide how you continue to prepare for the TEAS. If you feel you need more review and practice with human anatomy and physiology, you should study this chapter some more and use the online Qbank that comes with this book. After you have registered your book at **kaptest.com/booksonline**, log in to your student home page at **kaptest.com** to use your Qbank.

The TEAS also tests other areas of *Science*. In addition to asking questions about the skeletal, neuromuscular, and cardiovascular system, the TEAS assesses your knowledge of the other organ systems of the human body. The TEAS also asks questions about these topics:

- Biology and Chemistry
- Scientific Procedures and Reasoning

Lessons covering every human organ system, as well as the other *Science* concepts tested on the TEAS, will be included in Kaplan's *ATI TEAS*® *Strategies, Practice, & Review with 2 Practice Tests*, which will be available for purchase in early January 2017.

English and Language Usage

As a nursing or health science student and then later as a healthcare professional, you will be expected to express yourself clearly and correctly in writing. This skill will be important to your ability to communicate with clients and colleagues. You might be adding notes to a client's chart, writing out instructions for a client or colleague, or preparing educational material to distribute to clients or the public. The TEAS *English and language usage* content area tests your ability to use correct spelling, punctuation, and grammar; construct sentences and paragraphs to convey meaning clearly; and use appropriate vocabulary and style to communicate to a given audience.

Questions by Content Area

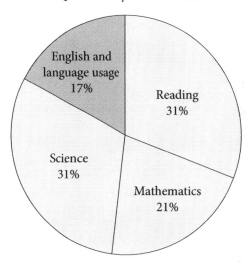

The TEAS English and Language Usage Content Area

Of the 170 items on the TEAS, 28 will be in the *English and language usage* content area, and you will have 28 minutes to answer them. This means you will have an average of 1 minute per question.

In the *English and language usage* section, 24 of the 28 questions will be scored, and 4 will be unscored. You won't know which questions are unscored, so do your best on every question.

The 24 scored *English and language usage* questions come from three sub-content areas:

Sub-content areas	# of Questions
Conventions of standard English	9
Knowledge of language	9
Vocabulary acquisition	6

Kaplan's *High-Yield Practice for the New ATI TEAS*® includes a chapter covering one of the areas of *English and language usage* that the TEAS tests most:

- Chapter 1: Spelling, Punctuation, and Sentence Structure

The Kaplan Method for English and Language Usage

Thinking through questions step-by-step will help you approach every question with the right rules in mind.

KAPLAN METHOD FOR ENGLISH AND LANGUAGE USAGE

Step 1: Analyze the information provided.

Step 2: Predict the answer.

Step 3: Evaluate the answer choices.

Step 1: Analyze the information provided.

Many questions about *English and language usage* will present you with a sentence or short passage and ask you to identify an element of the sentence, complete the sentence correctly, or fix an error. The question will specify what task you are to perform. Read the question and the sentence carefully, paying particular attention to the rule of grammar, spelling, punctuation, or style that you need to apply, as well as context clues in the sentence that point to the meaning of a word or its part of speech, a needed punctuation mark, or whatever you are being asked about.

Not every question is accompanied by a sentence. Some simply ask you to recall facts. In this case, the question still contains key terms that identify which fact you need to apply. The TEAS tests many language arts topics; you might see a question about writing style followed by one about punctuation followed by one about sentence structure. Each time you read a question, give yourself the time it takes for one deep breath to call to mind the particular rules or facts being tested.

Step 2: Predict the answer.

Before looking at the answer choices, *predict* the answer. You have a much better chance of finding the correct answer if you already have it in mind. Sometimes you may not be able to make a specific prediction. For example, a question might ask you to complete a sentence and there are several ways to complete the sentence correctly. Think of several ways you could complete the sentence and then use this mental checklist as you evaluate the answer choices.

Alternatively, you may have trouble thinking of the exact answer. Say the question asks for the part of a book that lists key terms alphabetically. You may not be able to think of the word *index* right off the bat, but you may know that you find such a list at the back of a book. Even an approximate prediction will allow you to eliminate answer choices you know are not found at the end of a book.

Step 3: Evaluate the answer choices.

Compare each answer choice to your prediction, eliminating those that are not a match and choosing the one that is a match.

SPELLING, PUNCTUATION, AND SENTENCE STRUCTURE

LEARNING OBJECTIVES

- Use standard English spelling conventions and common exceptions to these rules to spell words correctly
- Use punctuation correctly according to the standard rules of English
- Construct sentences with various structures and identify parts of speech and the main parts of sentences

Of the 24 scored *English and language usage* questions, 9 (37.5%) will be in the sub-content area of *Conventions of standard English*. The TEAS tests your recognition of and ability to use correct spelling, punctuation, and sentence structure.

This chapter addresses these skills in three lessons:

Lesson 1: Spelling

Lesson 2: Punctuation

Lesson 3: Sentence Structure

English and Language Usage Questions by Sub-content Area

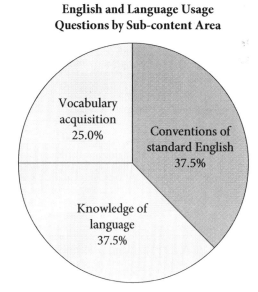

Vocabulary acquisition 25.0%

Conventions of standard English 37.5%

Knowledge of language 37.5%

LESSON 1

Spelling

LEARNING OBJECTIVES

- Spell words using standard English spelling conventions
- Identify common exceptions to standard English spelling conventions
- Recognize common words that have different meanings but are either spelled the same way (homographs) or sound the same (homophones)

English words come from different language families, all of which have rules that govern spelling. As a result, English spelling is notoriously difficult to master because most of its rules have multiple exceptions. Fortunately, the rules can be learned and their exceptions memorized!

Common Spelling Rules

You may recall learning the rhyme, "*i* before *e*, except after *c*," when you were a child. But you may not have learned that there is an easy way to remember additional exceptions to the "*i* before *e*" rule: if it sounds like a long a (as in *neighbor* or *weigh*), use *e* before *i*.

i before *e*	"After *c*" and "sounds like *a*" exceptions	Other exceptions
believe	ceiling	caffeine
chief	eight	neither
friend	receipt	protein
relief	vein	science
thief	weigh	weird

Many spelling errors occur when **suffixes** are added to words incorrectly. It is important to understand the rules and guidelines that dictate whether the endings of a **root word** should change when merged with a suffix; these are the Root Ends and Beginnings of Suffixes (REBS) rules. You may already know some of the REBS rules, but you should memorize any you do not recognize. You should also memorize the most common exceptions to these rules.

Word that . . .	Rule	Examples	Exceptions
ends in *e* + suffix beginning with a consonant	Keep the *e* if it is silent.	state + ment = statement peace + ful = peaceful encourage + ment = encouragement	judge + ment = judgment awe + ful = awful
ends in *e* + suffix beginning with a vowel	Drop the *e* if it is silent.	change + ing = changing shove + ing = shoving	Keep the *e* if the word ends in *ce, ge,* or *ke* and the suffix is *able* or *ous*. change + able = changeable outrage + ous = outrageous like + able = likeable
ends in *y* preceded by a consonant + suffix	Change the *y* to *i* and add the suffix.	carry + er = carrier duty + ful = dutiful worry + ed = worried	Keep the *y* when adding the suffix *ing*. carry + ing = carrying rely + ing = relying worry + ing = worrying
ends in *ay, ey, oy, uy* + any suffix	Keep the *y*.	relay + ed = relayed survey + ing = surveying destroy + er = destroyer buy + er = buyer	
ends in a consonant-vowel-consonant and is only one syllable + suffix beginning with a vowel	Double the final consonant and add the suffix.	scrub + ing = scrubbing tag + ed = tagged run + ing = running knit + ed = knitted	Omit the double consonant if the word ends in *w*. sew + ing = sewing snow + ed = snowed blow + ing = blowing
ends in a consonant-vowel-consonant but has more than one syllable (and the last syllable is stressed) + suffix beginning with a vowel	Double the final consonant and add the suffix.	control + ing = controlling defer + al = deferral refer + ed = referred occur + ing = occurring	Omit the double consonant if the word ends in *w*. renew + ing = renewing

Word that . . .	Rule	Examples	Exceptions
ends in *c* + suffix beginning with *e, i,* or *y*	Add a *k* then add the suffix.	panic + ed = panicked frolic + ing = frolicking garlic + y = garlicky	

Here is how an expert would answer a TEAS question that tests a spelling rule.

Question	Analysis
Sharla ate a _____ bar on her way to the meeting.	**Step 1**: You need to find the correctly spelled word that fills the blank in the sentence.
Which of the following correctly completes the sentence above?	**Step 2**: You cannot predict the word that will fill the blank. However, a glance at the answer choices tells you that spelling rules are involved, so call to mind the rules you know.
(A) proteen	**Step 3**: Is this the correct spelling of *protein*? No.
(B) protien	Is this the correct spelling of *protein*? No.
(C) protein	Is this the correct spelling of *protein*? Yes. This word is an exception to the *i* before *e* rule.
(D) protine	This is not the correct spelling of *protein*.

Now try a question that tests a different rule.

Which of the following is spelled correctly?
- (A) defered
- (B) occurred
- (C) patroled
- (D) snowwing

Explanation

Step 1: You need to find the correctly spelled word.

Step 2: With this type of question, you cannot predict which word will be correctly spelled, but you can call to mind the spelling rules you have memorized. Then evaluate each answer choice and determine which one correctly fills the blank.

Step 3: Answer choice **(B)** obeys the REBS rule for doubling the final consonant before adding a suffix: occur + ed = occurred.

Making Singular Words Plural

Other spelling rules you should be familiar with relate to the formation of plurals. Most of the time, simply adding s to the end of a singular word creates the correct plural form: *peanut* becomes *peanuts*, for example. However, there are rules about when you need to do something different to create a plural. The table lists some of the common rules for forming plurals that you might see tested on the TEAS.

Word that . . .	Rule	Examples	Exceptions
ends in a consonant other than *s, x, y, z, ch*, or *sh*	Add *s*.	cat/cats dog/dogs owl/owls	
ends in *s, x, ch*, or *sh*	Add *es*.	bus/buses box/boxes church/churches wish/wishes	axis/axes ox/oxen appendix/appendixes or appendices
ends in *z*	Double the *z* and add *es*.	quiz/quizzes	
ends in *y* preceded by a vowel	Add *s*.	holiday/holidays monkey/monkeys	money/monies
ends in *y* preceded by a consonant	Change the *y* to *i* and add *es*.	baby/babies story/stories	
ends in *f* or *fe*	Change the *f* to *v* and add *es*.	calf/calves leaf/leaves	chief/chiefs proof/proofs
ends in a vowel	Add *s*.	coffee/coffees sale/sales taco/tacos	potato/potatoes veto/vetoes

Learning these rules and the common exceptions will give you an edge on the TEAS *English and language usage* test.

Homonyms

Words that are spelled the same way but have different meanings are called **homographs**. Those that sound alike but have different spellings and meanings are called **homophones**. Together, homographs and homophones are called **homonyms**. The table lists some homographs, homophones, and other commonly confused words that people often misspell or misuse.

Word	Meaning	Word in sentence
accept	to receive willingly	I accept your apology.
except	excluding	They were all present except Lara, who stayed home.
affect	to impact	The gray weather affects my mood.
effect	a result	The drug's effects will wear off soon.
content	something contained	The book's content is very disturbing.
	at peace or soothed	The baby was content in her mother's arms.
close	nearby	His house is close to his birthplace.
	to shut	Close the door, please.
clothes	apparel	I would like to change clothes first.
desert	arid land	I've never been to the desert.
	to leave behind	You said you would never desert me.
dessert	sweet food served after a meal	A good hostess offers dessert to her guests.
fare	money paid for transportation	She paid her subway fare in nickels.
fair	just or right	It was only fair that he let you go first.
	a festival	After all, it was your first trip to the fair.
forth	forward	Go forth and seek adventure!
fourth	in the 4th position	Her house is the fourth one on the left.
grate	to shred	We will need to grate some cheese before serving the pasta.
great	fabulous, fantastic	This will be a great dinner!
	of large size	We will eat in the great hall.
hole	an opening	This sweater has a hole in it.
whole	entire, entirety	I can't believe I ate the whole thing.
its	possessive form of the pronoun *it*	The turtle ducked into its shell.
it's	contraction of *it is*	It's freezing in here!
led	past tense of the verb *lead*	He led the visitors to the cafeteria after the tour.
lead	a metal; the material in pencils	My pencil is out of lead.
	to guide or bring forward	The captain should lead the charge.

Word	Meaning	Word in sentence
lessen	to reduce or decrease	Hopefully this will lessen the pain a bit.
lesson	something you learn or teach	Next time he will have learned his lesson.
passed	went by	Have you passed the post office yet?
past	opposite of *future*	I lived there in the past but not now.
principal	head of a school	The principal will meet with the seniors.
	primary, most significant	Cost was the principal reason she cited when explaining the decision.
principle	a guiding rule	Failing to act would violate my principles.
their	belonging to them	That is their car.
there	at that place, opposite of *here*	The car is parked over there.
they're	contraction of *they are*	They're going to try to sell it.
to	indicates direction	Please go to the store for me.
too	also, in addition	Erika will go, too.
two	the number 2	Buy two loaves of bread.
weak	the opposite of *strong*	Having the flu has left me feeling weak.
week	seven days	I have been sick since last week.
your	possessive form of *you*	Don't forget your mittens!
you're	contraction of *you are*	You're going to need them on the way home.

Here is how an expert would answer a question about homonyms.

Question	Analysis
The teacher had prepared his lessons for the week, but on Monday mourning, he was late arriving at school because the bus had passed his house without stopping.	**Step 1:** There are several homophones in this sentence, so these are likely places for an error.
Which of the following describes the error in the sentence above?	**Step 2:** Assess the homophones to determine which one is incorrect; *mourning* means sorrow or bereavement and does not work in this sentence. Predict that the correct word here is *morning*, which is a time of day.

Question	Analysis
(A) The word *lessons* should be *lessens*.	**Step 3**: *Lessons* is the correct word in this sentence.
(B) The word *week* should be *weak*.	*Week* is the correct word in this sentence.
(C) The word *mourning* should be *morning*.	Correct. This matches your prediction.
(D) The word *passed* should be *past*.	*Passed*, the past tense of the verb *pass*, is the correct word for this sentence.

KEY IDEAS

- English spelling is governed by rules, but most of these rules have common exceptions.
- Spelling errors commonly occur where word roots meet suffixes, including plurals. Learn the rules and the common exceptions to spot these errors quickly.
- Homophones and homographs are easily confused, so make flashcards with any that give you trouble.

Spelling Practice Questions

1. Which of the following words is spelled incorrectly?

   (A) Permissible
   (B) Disbelief
   (C) Wierd
   (D) Judgment

2. Consuming too much salt can be _____ to your health.

   Which of the following correctly completes the sentence above?

   (A) injuryious
   (B) injurieous
   (C) injurrious
   (D) injurious

3. The fawn _____ beside the pond, unaware that we were watching.

   Which of the following correctly completes the sentence above?

   (A) frolicked
   (B) frolicced
   (C) froliced
   (D) frolicted

4. The _____ reason he gave for refusing to wear leather shoes was that doing so violated his _____ as a strict vegetarian.

   Select the pair of homophones that correctly completes the sentence above.

   (A) principle/principals
   (B) principal/principles
   (C) principle/principles
   (D) principal/principals

Review your work using the explanations in Part Six of this book.

LESSON 2

Punctuation

LEARNING OBJECTIVES

- Recognize the three sentence punctuation patterns
- Use end punctuation marks and commas to clarify meaning
- Use colons, semicolons, apostrophes, and parentheses correctly within a sentence
- Use direct and indirect quotations according to the standard rules of English

Punctuation is an essential component of written language. These unassuming marks and symbols play a huge role—giving structure and clarity to the ideas expressed in writing and allowing authors to relate meaning, ask questions, identify direct quotations, and emphasize particular ideas or facts.

Sentence Punctuation Patterns

Punctuation organizes ideas into sentences, which can be characterized as having one of three primary punctuation patterns—simple, complex, or compound.

A **simple sentence** contains only one clause and has a single subject and predicate. The predicate contains the verb and tells us something about the subject.

> *Example:* We divided up the chores.

A **complex sentence** contains both an independent and a dependent, or subordinate, clause. An independent clause has both a subject and a verb and expresses a complete thought. A dependent clause also has a subject and a verb but does not express a complete thought.

> *Example:* Although I ran the marathon last spring, I will not be running it again this year.

A **compound sentence** contains at least two independent clauses, which are connected by either a coordinating conjunction and a comma or a semicolon.

> *Example:* I purchased two tickets to the show, but I am no longer able to attend.

Being able to distinguish the different sentence punctuation patterns is essential to success on the TEAS. The type of sentence pattern determines the type of punctuation required within the sentence.

End Punctuation Marks

End punctuation marks tell the reader the purpose of the sentence. A period indicates a declarative sentence that describes something, states information, or gives a command. A question mark indicates a question. The exclamation point indicates a sentence that expresses strong emotions or excitement.

Comma Usage

The comma is one of the most commonly used punctuation marks. When used correctly, the comma helps the reader understand how ideas in a sentence are connected. There are numerous rules that govern comma usage, and the TEAS may test any of the those listed in the table.

Comma Usage	
Usage guideline or rule	**Example**
Commas can indicate a pause, such as after introductory information.	*Before the development of Portland cement,* architects rarely used concrete block construction.
Commas can present phrases that are not essential to the meaning of the sentence.	Asha, *who is a straight A student,* attends Roosevelt High.
Commas are used to show a direct address, or calling a person by name.	*Jake,* please put the roast in the oven.
Commas can separate items in a list.	Jodi put *bananas, pears, and oranges* in the fruit salad.
Commas divide a series of words, phrases, or clauses.	Today we will *drive to swim practice, stop at the grocery store, and make dinner.*
Commas can separate adjectives that both describe a word equally. If you can separate the adjectives with *and*, then a comma is usually appropriate.	Pete visited the *old, crumbling* house one last time. Pete visited the *big green* house one last time. (no comma)
Commas follow the salutation and the closing in an informal letter or note.	Dear *Jaden,* I can't wait to see you. *Love,* Mom
Do *not* use a comma to set off an essential phrase. Essential phrases often include the word *that.*	Monika ate the cake *that Annie made for her.*
Commas are used to separate the elements in dates and place names.	June 12, 1979 Detroit, Michigan

Let's now see how a test expert would tackle a question dealing with commas.

Question	Analysis
Which of the following is a correctly punctuated compound sentence?	**Step 1:** The question asks you to identify a correctly punctuated compound sentence, and the answer choices are four sentences.
	Step 2: The correct answer will consist of two independent clauses joined by either a comma and coordinating conjunction or a semicolon.

Question	Analysis
(A) After school lets out the children will go to the park.	**Step 3**: This is a complex sentence, and a comma is missing after "out." Eliminate.
(B) All of the children rode their bikes to school, so they will ride to the park as well.	Correct. This sentence has two independent clauses that are correctly connected by a coordinating conjunction and a comma.
(C) The weather is warm, they need to drink enough water to stay hydrated.	This sentence has two independent clauses connected by a comma, but the coordinating conjunction is missing. Eliminate.
(D) Before they go home for dinner; the children will go down the slide one more time.	This sentence is a complex sentence that incorrectly uses a semicolon in the place of a comma. Eliminate.

Colons, Semicolons, Apostrophes, and Parentheses

Familiarize yourself with the rules associated with these punctuation marks.

Common Punctuation Marks

Punctuation Mark	Usage	Example
colon	A punctuation mark signaling a list or information that adds to the idea before the colon. Colons may also be used after the salutation in formal letters or memos.	My mother told me to buy the following: a loaf of bread, a container of milk, and a stick of butter. To whom it may concern: Dear Sir or Madam:
semicolon	A punctuation mark used to link related independent clauses or a series of items containing commas	The cello player forgot her music; therefore, she had to improvise during her performance. For their picnic, Michael purchased apples, bananas, and grapes; Jana bought bread, cheese, and jam; and Julian picked up lemonade and ice tea.
apostrophe	A punctuation mark used to form possessives and contractions and to pluralize letters, numbers, or other words that have no plural form	Jim's golf clubs, Rosa's house Dot your *i*'s and cross your *t*'s!
parentheses	Punctuation marks used to enclose additional information or explanations that would interrupt the flow of the sentence.	Karyn will (I assume) remember to bring the potato salad.

Let's see how a test expert would tackle a question testing these punctuation rules.

Question	Analysis
The librarian tried repeatedly to quiet the noisy children, but she was unsuccessful; eventually, she took each childs' book away and escorted the rowdy group to the lobby. Which of the following punctuation marks is used incorrectly in the sentence?	**Step 1:** The question asks about punctuation. A sentence is given with two commas, a semicolon, an apostrophe, and an ending period. Examine each in terms of the rules for that mark.
	Step 2: The word "child" is singular; therefore, the apostrophe should come before the "s" in the possessive form.
(A) The comma after the word "children"	**Step 3:** This is a compound sentence, in which the comma correctly comes before the coordinating conjunction that separates the two independent clauses. Eliminate.
(B) The semicolon after the word "unsuccessful"	The semicolon correctly separates two independent clauses in this sentence. Eliminate.
(C) The comma after the word "eventually"	The comma correctly separates the introductory adverb "eventually" from the rest of the sentence. Eliminate.
(D) The apostrophe in the word childs'	Correct.

Punctuation for Quotations

Written dialogue represents the exact language someone has used when speaking. For example, a nurse may need to quote a patient's exact words to include on intake or medical reports. When writing a quote, the rules of using quotation marks apply.

Quotation Marks and Dialogue Rules	
Rule	**Example**
Quotation marks must come in pairs. If you open a quotation mark, it must be closed at the end of the quote.	"Always remember to close the quote," the teacher said.
Capitalize the first letter of a direct quote if the quote represents a complete sentence.	Danny said, "You never told me it was your birthday!"
Do not capitalize the first letter of a direct quote if it is a fragment or incomplete sentence.	Jamie said the new car was "the cat's meow."
Do not capitalize the second part of a quote if it is interrupted midsentence.	"I don't know what it was," said Peter, "but it sure was big!"
Enclose a comma before closing the quote prior to attribution.	"I've never tried chop suey before," said Katie.

Quotation Marks and Dialogue Rules

Rule	Example
A quote within a quote takes single quotation marks.	"And then she said, 'No way!' as she huffed off," Erin told me.
Short works such as chapters, songs, poems, and short stories should have their titles enclosed in quotation marks.	We read "Ode on a Grecian Urn" in our English class.
The ending punctuation mark for the quote should be enclosed within the quotation marks. Use a comma to transition from quote to attribution.	Jerry said, "All's well that ends well." "She gave me the best present," said Karen.

Let's see how a test expert would approach the following question.

Question	Analysis
Which of the following sentences correctly punctuates the direct dialogue?	**Step 1:** The question asks about punctuating direct dialogue, and the answer choices are four sentences within quotation marks. Evaluate each sentence in terms of the rules for quotation marks, commas, and capitalization in dialogue.
	Step 2: Mentally review the applicable rules and prepare to check each answer choice against them. When you see an answer has broken a rule, you can stop reading it and eliminate it.
(A) "Whenever the teacher wants the students' attention, she calls out "Silence!" to the class," said the principal.	**Step 3:** This sentence fails to include the comma after the attribution to the teacher, and it uses double quotation marks within the principal's quote. Eliminate.
(B) "Whenever the teacher wants the students' attention, she calls out, 'Silence!' to the class," said the principal.	Correct.
(C) "Whenever the teacher wants the students' attention, she calls out, "silence!" to the class." Said the principal.	This sentence fails to capitalize the first letter of "silence," it closes the quote with a period rather than a comma, and it has double quotation marks within the principal's quote. Eliminate.
(D) "Whenever the teacher wants the students' attention, she calls out 'silence!' to the class," said the principal.	This sentence fails to include the comma after the attribution to the teacher, and it fails to capitalize the first letter of "silence." Eliminate.

KEY IDEAS

- Learning the three different sentence punctuation patterns will help you recognize punctuation errors on the TEAS.

- Analyze the content and structure of a sentence to determine which end punctuation is needed and where commas belong.

- Examine the structure of a sentence to determine whether colons, semicolons, apostrophes, and parentheses are either misplaced or incorrectly omitted.

- If a sentence contains a direct quotation, check that it follows standard English rules for capitalization and the placement of quotation marks, commas, and end punctuation.

Punctuation Practice Questions

1. Which of the following is a correctly punctuated complex sentence?

   (A) Every weekend in the summer Daniel goes hiking on a mountain trail.
   (B) Daniel usually hikes alone, however, this time he invited me to join him.
   (C) Although I am an experienced hiker, I was not prepared for the rocky terrain.
   (D) I was relieved, when we reached the summit and could stop to enjoy the view.

2. Which of the following examples is a correct method for punctuating this quotation?

   (A) "We must all do our part" she said, "even when doing so is difficult."
   (B) "We must all do our part," she said, "even when doing so is difficult."
   (C) "We must all do our part." She said, "even when doing so is difficult."
   (D) "We must all do our part," she said. "even when doing so is difficult."

3. Which of the following sentences is correctly punctuated?

   (A) Because the weather forecast predicted storms we decided to postpone our vacation until next month.
   (B) Because the weather forecast predicted storms. We decided to postpone our vacation until next month.
   (C) Because the weather forecast predicted storms; we decided to postpone our vacation until next month.
   (D) Because the weather forecast predicted storms, we decided to postpone our vacation until next month.

4. Veronica has performed well on every test she has taken this semester_____therefore, she can expect to perform well on the final exam.

   Which of the following punctuation marks best completes the sentence?

   (A) .
   (B) ;
   (C) ,
   (D) :

Review your work using the explanations in Part Six of this book.

LESSON 3

Sentence Structure

LEARNING OBJECTIVES

- Identify the correct use of eight parts of speech
- Construct simple, compound, complex, and compound-complex sentences
- Construct sentences using dependent and independent clauses
- Identify the main parts of sentence structures

Eight Parts of Speech

The eight parts of speech defined here are the most commonly tested parts of speech on the TEAS.

noun	a person, place, or thing
pronoun	a word (such as *I, he, she, you, it, we,* or *they*) that is used instead of a noun
verb	a word (such as *jump, think, happen,* or *exist*) that expresses an action or state of being
adjective	a word (such as *funny, breakable,* or *round*) that describes a noun or a pronoun
adverb	a word (such as *quickly, cheerfully,* or *very*) used to modify a verb, adjective, or another adverb
preposition	a word expressing a relationship to other words (such as *on* in "the drawing on the page" and *after* in "she arrived after the play")
conjunction	a word used to connect clauses or sentences (such as *and, but,* or *if*)
interjection	a word or phrase that expresses sudden or strong feeling (such as *Hooray!* or *Oh!*)

Here is how an expert would answer a TEAS question about parts of speech.

Question	Analysis
Holland laughed loudly when he heard the joke. What are the noun and pronoun pair in the sentence above?	**Step 1:** The question asks you to identify the noun and pronoun in the sentence, and the answer choices list pairs of words from the sentence.
	Step 2: A noun is a person, place, or thing, and a pronoun is a word used instead of a noun. The noun/pronoun pair in this sentence is "Holland/he."

Question	Analysis
(A) Noun: he; pronoun: Holland	**Step 3:** This reverses the noun and pronoun. Eliminate.
(B) Noun: Holland; pronoun: laughed	This gets the noun correct but incorrectly identifies the verb "laughed" as the pronoun. Eliminate.
(C) Noun: he; pronoun: laughed	Here the pronoun is incorrectly identified as the noun, and a verb is used as the pronoun. Eliminate.
(D) Noun: Holland; pronoun: he	Correct. This matches the prediction.

Now try a question on your own.

> The ballerina danced beautifully despite her broken shoe and torn tutu.
>
> What are the verb and adverb in the sentence above?
>
> (A) Verb: ballerina; adverb: her
> (B) Verb: danced; adverb: despite
> (C) Verb: danced; adverb: beautifully
> (D) Verb: broken; adverb: shoe

Explanation

Step 1: The question asks you to identify the verb and adverb in the sentence, and the answer choices list pairs of words from the sentence.

Step 2: A verb is a word that expresses an action or state of being, and an adverb is a word used to modify a verb, adjective, or another adverb. The verb in this sentence is "danced," and the adverb is "beautifully," telling how she danced.

Step 3: Answer choice **(C)** matches the prediction.

Simple, Compound, Complex, and Compound-Complex Sentences

To be complete, a **simple sentence** must have at least one subject and one verb, and it must express a complete thought. The **subject** is the main noun of the sentence that is doing or being. The verb tells what action the subject is doing. These simple sentences are also called independent clauses.

> *Example:* Scarlett attended the training.

 "Scarlett" is the subject, and "attended" is the verb.

Two or more independent clauses can be joined in a **compound sentence.** A compound sentence gives the ideas in the two clauses equal weight. To make a compound sentence, choose a coordinating conjunction (*for, and, nor, but, or, yet, so*) to join the independent clauses and insert a comma before the conjunction. Only these conjunctions can form compound sentences. Use the acronym FANBOYS to help you remember the conjunctions: For, And, Nor, But, Or, Yet, and So.

> *Example:* Scarlett attended the training, so she knows the protocol.

 "Scarlett attended the training" is an independent clause, and "she knows the protocol" is also an independent clause. "So" is a coordinating conjunction joining the two clauses.

A **complex sentence** combines an independent clause with a dependent clause. A dependent clause has a subject and verb, but it does not express a complete thought. Another term for *dependent clause* is *subordinate clause.* The idea in the dependent clause provides additional information to support the idea in the independent clause.

> *Example:* Scarlett attended the training because it was required.

The independent clause is still "Scarlett attended the training," but now there is a dependent clause, "because it was required." On its own, "Because it was required," would be a sentence fragment instead of a complete sentence.

Compound-complex sentences incorporate two independent clauses and one or more dependent clauses. An independent clause contains a subject and verb and expresses a complete thought. A dependent clause contains a subject and verb but does not express a complete thought, so it cannot be a sentence.

> *Example:* Because it was required, Scarlett attended the training, so now she knows the protocol.

Once again, "Scarlett attended the training" is an independent clause, but now it is joined to another independent clause and accompanied by a dependent clause.

Here is how an expert would answer a TEAS question that tests a rule about sentence types.

Question	Analysis
Which of the following is a simple sentence?	**Step 1**: The question asks you to identify a simple sentence, and the answer choices are four sentences.
	Step 2: A simple sentence contains a subject and a verb and expresses a complete thought.
(A) Driving all the way to the country.	**Step 3**: This is not a complete sentence. It is a sentence fragment. Eliminate.
(B) The car that needed gasoline.	This is also not a complete sentence. Eliminate.
(C) The car needed gasoline because they were driving all the way to the country.	Because two clauses are joined with "because," this is a complex sentence. Eliminate.
(D) The car needs gasoline for the drive to the country.	Correct. This is a simple sentence that uses a subject and a verb and expresses a complete thought. Note that "for" is not used as a coordinating conjunction here because "the drive to the country" is not an independent clause.

Now you try one.

> Which of the following would NOT complete the sentence correctly with a dependent clause?
>
> She didn't want to drink the coffee, _____.
>
> > (A)   because it was very hot
> > (B)   although she was not in a hurry
> > (C)   and neither did I
> > (D)   since breakfast wasn't ready yet

Explanation

Step 1: The question asks you to choose the one answer choice that does *not* complete the sentence correctly with a dependent clause, and the answer choices list independent and dependent clauses.

Step 2: A dependent clause contains a subject and verb but does not express a complete thought. The correct answer here will *not* be a dependent clause. It may be an independent clause or a fragment (phrase).

Step 3: Only answer choice **(C)**, beginning with "and," is not a dependent clause. It expresses a complete thought (*I didn't want to drink the coffee either*) and could stand alone as a sentence. The other answer choices are dependent clauses and could not stand alone.

Parts of Sentences

Knowing other sentence parts will help you analyze sentence structures that are tested on the TEAS. Here are additional terms that you need to know.

Part of Sentence	Definition
subject	the person or thing that is performing the action or being described
object	a person or thing that receives the action of the verb
indirect object	a person or thing to whom/which or for whom/which something is done
predicate	the part of a sentence that expresses what a subject does
complement	a word or group of words added to a sentence to make it complete
article	a word (such as *a*, *an*, or *the*) used with a noun to limit it or make it clearer
modifier	a word (such as an adjective or adverb) or phrase that describes another word or group of words

Example: The girl happily read him the book. It was funny.

In the first sentence, "The girl" is the complete subject, and "happily read him the book" is the complete predicate. "The" is an article, and "happily" is a modifier (an adverb telling how she read). "The book" is the object of her reading, and "him" is the indirect object.

In the second sentence, "It" is the subject, and "was funny" is the complete predicate. "Funny" is a complement because "It was," though consisting of a noun and a verb, would not form a sentence that made sense.

Here is how a test expert would answer a TEAS question that tests the parts of sentence structure.

Question	Analysis
She gave me the chocolate. Which of the following correctly identifies the direct object and indirect object of the sentence?	**Step 1:** This simple sentence includes the subject "She," the verb "gave," the direct object "chocolate," and the indirect object "me." The question asks about the two kinds of objects.
	Step 2: The correct answer will identify "chocolate" as the direct object and "me" as the indirect object.
(A) Direct: me; indirect: She	**Step 3:** Incorrectly identifies the indirect object "me" as the direct object and incorrectly identifies the subject "She" as the indirect object. Eliminate.
(B) Direct: She; indirect: me	Incorrectly identifies the subject "She" as the direct object, although it gets the indirect object right. Eliminate.
(C) Direct: chocolate; indirect: me	This matches the prediction. Correct.
(D) Direct: chocolate; indirect: She	Incorrectly identifies the subject "She" as the indirect object. Eliminate.

KEY IDEAS

- Knowing the eight parts of speech and the parts of sentences (such as subject, predicate, object, indirect object, complement) is key to analyzing sentence structure.
- An independent clause could stand alone as a simple sentence. A dependent clause cannot stand alone.
- You can distinguish among simple, compound, complex, and compound-complex sentences by whether they include independent and/or dependent clauses and how the clauses are connected.

Sentence Structure Practice Questions

1. Working hard is important if you want to achieve your goals.

   Which of the following is the subject of the independent clause in the sentence above?

   (A) Working
   (B) important
   (C) you
   (D) goals

2. Bob was generous in his praise of Gil's pleasant nature.

   Which of the following is the pronoun in the sentence above?

   (A) Bob
   (B) generous
   (C) his
   (D) nature

3. Which of the following is an example of a compound-complex sentence?

   (A) Because the book was confusing, Sarah stopped reading it, so now she needs something new to read.
   (B) Sarah stopped reading the most confusing book she had ever encountered.
   (C) Sarah stopped reading the book immediately when it started confusing her.
   (D) Sarah immediately stopped reading the confusing book.

4. He told me a very long and boring story.

   Which of the following is the direct object in the sentence above?

   (A) He
   (B) me
   (C) boring
   (D) story

Review your work using the explanations in Part Six of this book.

Review and Reflect

Think about the questions you answered in these lessons.

- Were you able to approach each question systematically, using the Kaplan Method for English and Language Usage?
- If one or more sentences were provided, were you able to analyze them efficiently, identifying clues to the correct answer?
- Did you feel confident that you understood what the question was asking you to do?
- How well were you able to predict an answer before looking at the answer choices?
- Could you match your prediction to the correct answer?
- Are there areas of language arts that appear on the TEAS that you don't understand as well as you would like?
- If you missed any questions, do you understand why the answer you chose is incorrect and why the right answer is correct? Could you do the question again now and get it right?

Use your thoughts about these questions to guide how you continue to prepare for the TEAS. If you feel you need more review and practice with spelling, punctuation, and sentence structure, you should study this chapter some more and use the online Qbank that comes with this book. After you have registered your book at **kaptest.com/booksonline**, log in to your student home page at **kaptest.com** to use your Qbank.

The TEAS also tests two other areas of *English and language usage*:

- Grammar, Style, and the Writing Process
- Vocabulary

Chapters with lessons addressing these concepts and skills will be included in Kaplan's *ATI TEAS*® *Strategies, Practice, & Review with 2 Practice Tests,* which will be available for purchase in early January 2017.

Answers and Explanations

In this part of your book, you will find answers and explanations for every set of practice questions at the end of the lessons.

Even if you got a question correct, you may still learn something from the explanation. Therefore, review all of the explanations carefully. If you missed a question, first read the explanation to understand why you missed it. Then try that question again in a few days or a week to make sure you still remember how to do it. While reading about how you could have done a question correctly is helpful, actually doing the question correctly is an even more effective way of reinforcing your learning.

As you review, keep track of both your strengths and areas where you would like to improve. Use your performance to determine where you will focus your study time so you can maximize your score on the TEAS.

Good luck!

Reading Answers and Explanations

Chapter 1: Main Ideas and Supporting Details

Lesson 1: Strategic Reading

Questions 1–6: Passage Map

Topic: Urban legends
Scope: What they are
Purpose: Inform
¶ 1: Urban legend = modern folktale, not true
¶ 2: Example—alligators in sewers
¶ 3: Example—kidney removal; ULs sometimes widely believed

1. **(B) urban legends.** The topic, urban legends, is introduced in the first sentence, and the rest of the passage provides more information about them and two examples, making choice **(B)** correct. Choices (A) and (C) are details about urban legends, and choice (D) is a detail from the example showing how they change.

2. **(D) a basis in reality.** This is an EXCEPT detail question, so the correct answer is the one that does *not* characterize successful urban legends. Because you can't find something that isn't there, research the answer choices one by one and eliminate those that are stated in the passage. The author calls urban legends "folktales" and "stories," which means that they're fictional, leaving **(D)** as the correct answer. All other answers are in paragraph 1.

3. **(A) Their themes change with the times.** This question is about a specific claim made in the passage, so it is a detail question. The first sentence of the third paragraph states that urban legends change over time, matching choice **(A)**. Choice (B) is the opposite of what the passage says; most urban legends cannot be verified. Choice (C) is also an opposite, since urban legends have emerged "in modern society." Choice (D) contradicts the information in the last sentence that urban legends are mainly transmitted "through emails and social media."

4. **(C) a new form of folklore.** The author's primary concern is the topic of the passage. The entire passage is about urban legends, so predict that as the topic and match it with answer choice **(C).** Choices (A) and (B) are details from two legends, and choice (D) refers to a word in the third paragraph, another detail.

5. **(D) aligned with popular beliefs.** The phrase "according to the passage" always signals a detail question, and the answer is directly stated in the passage. In the first paragraph, the author writes that urban legends "persist . . . for the transmission of popular values and beliefs." Another way of saying this is that the legends are compatible, or align with, popular beliefs. Thus, choice **(D)** is correct. Choice (A) is out of scope; though "urban" means "city," the author never says urban legends persist in cities only. Choice (B) is the opposite of the information in the passage, and (C) is extreme in its use of the word "never." Certainly some people believe urban legends or they wouldn't tell them over and over.

6. **(B) All urban legends instill fear in listeners.** Like question 2, this asks for a detail that is not in the passage. Again, research the answer choices and eliminate those that are stated in the passage. Having done this, you are left with choice **(B).** Choice (A) is in paragraph 2, (C) is in paragraph 3, and (D) is in paragraph 1.

Lesson 2: Reading for Details

Questions 1–2: Passage Map

Topic: Basis of life
Scope: Sun/photosynthesis important to most, but not all life
Purpose: Inform
¶ 1: Life not dependent on sun was considered very rare
¶ 2: Recent discoveries: Whole ecosystems not dependent on sun

1. **(D) Sunlight** The first sentence states that "[m]ost life is fundamentally dependent on organisms that store radiant energy from the Sun." That's a longer way of saying "most life depends ultimately on sunlight." The photosynthetic plants and algae of choice (A) ultimately derive their energy from the sun, while sub-sea ecosystems (B) and chemosynthetic bacteria (C) refer to details that only concern research into deep-sea life.

2. **(A) Both are at the base of their respective food chains.** The first paragraph describes ecosystems that are dependent on photosynthetic organisms, while the second paragraph describes ecosystems that are dependent on chemosynthetic organisms. In both cases, though, the organisms serve similar functions as primary producers at the base of their different food chains. Choice (B) is incorrect because only chemosynthetic organisms are described as dependent on

energy from within the Earth. Choice (C) is incorrect because according to the passage, chemosynthetic organisms get their energy from the Earth, not sunlight. The relative numbers of these organisms, choice (D), is never discussed in the passage.

3. **(B) 2** According to the timeline, only *Queen Nofretete* and *Nike of Samothrace* are dated before the Common Era (BCE). All the other artwork dates have no postscript, which by convention means the dates are of the Common Era.

4. **(A) *Nike of Samothrace* and Lindisfarne Gospels** The timeline indicates that the *Nike of Samothrace* and the Lindisfarne Gospels are separated by nine centuries, making **(A)** the correct choice. The artworks in choice (B), *Arnolfini Wedding Portrait* and *Mrs. Siddons,* are also separated by centuries, but the gap is only about 350 years. Both choice (C), *Robie House* and *Girl Before a Mirror,* and choice (D), *The Scream* and *Robie House,* feature artworks separated by only a few decades and can be quickly eliminated.

5. **(D) Gettysburg** The map indicates that the Battle of Gettysburg took place in Pennsylvania. Gettysburg is further north than choice (A), First Battle of Bull Run, Virginia; (B), Antietam, Maryland; and (C), Shiloh, Tennessee.

6. **(C) West Virginia** Referring to the map's legend, you can see that West Virginia was a slave state that remained loyal to the Union. Choice (A), Texas, joined the Confederacy, choice (B), Arizona, was a territory during this period, and choice (D), Ohio, was a free state.

Lesson 3: Making Inferences

Questions 1–5: Passage Map

Topic: Arizona Desert products
Scope: Robe and blanket—benefits
Purpose: Sell the products
¶ 1: Have economy + comfort w/AD products
¶ 2: Blanket, robe keep you warm
¶ 3: Easy to maintain & safe

1. **(A) an advertising brochure.** The tone of the passage is very sales-like. You can infer that it is meant to convince a generic person to purchase this product and is not addressed to a specific person, as a personal email, (D), would be. Sales material, like advertising copy from a brochure, is written to tout the benefits of a product, not provide an objective evaluation as a consumer magazine, (B), or government report, (C), would try to do.

2. **(B) consumers who use Arizona Desert products will lower their heating costs.** You're looking for an idea that can be inferred but is not directly stated. Despite the comparison to a toaster, we know this blanket is meant to warm people up, not toast bread. It's the power consumption that is similar (less than 15 cents per day). But although this sounds inexpensive, it doesn't explain how the blanket could pay for itself unless it creates cost savings somewhere else. We can infer, then, that consumers using this blanket will not run their heating as much, and using the blanket will cost less than heating the home. The passage certainly implies that cost is an important consideration for consumers, so choice (D) is not supported.

3. **(B) air conditioners use more energy than fans.** In the first paragraph, the author compares noisy fans and energy-hogging air conditioners. It's implied that each alternative for staying cool has its own drawbacks. From this, you can reasonably infer that an air-conditioning unit is not loud relative to a fan, and a fan is low in its energy usage compared to an air conditioner. Therefore, choice **(B)** is correct. Choice (A) is not supported by the passage. Choice (C) contradicts the implication that the company has been around for some time, having at least one well-established product and one it has just released. Choice (D) might seem reasonable at first glance, but the beginning of the second paragraph implies that people use electric blankets in order to turn down their central heating, not because they don't have any. In fact, in cold parts of the country, central heating is generally not considered optional.

4. **(D) Country of manufacture.** The passage's author makes a point of mentioning (C) comfort, (A) the energy usage or energy cost of the blanket and robe relative to regular household heating, and even (B) safety, when noting there is no danger of contact with the chemical fluid. We can infer that the author, who appears to be writing advertising copy, believes these factors to be important to a person making a consumer decision. The author never mentions country of manufacture, so it's also reasonable to infer that he considers this less important than the other three factors.

5 **(C) Choking hazard—do not swallow.** The passage does not say anything about warning labels, but you can infer the answer based on information in the passage concerning safety. The third paragraph states that "you are never exposed to any risk" from the chemical fluid. This strongly implies that the chemical would not be safe if you were to break open the tubes and spill it or drink it. It would be appropriate to note its toxicity on a warning label, (A). You know from the first paragraph that this is an electric blanket (or robe), so a warning not to submerge it in water is reasonable, (B). The warning in the last paragraph to return the blanket right away if it

malfunctions or is damaged and not to replace or repair parts yourself also suggests danger, so this is likely to end up on a warning label (D). Only answer choice (C) is not supported. These products are a blanket and robe large enough to cover an adult. There is no reference to small, detachable parts that a person could conceivably swallow, so there is no evidence of a choking hazard.

Lesson 4: Understanding Sequences of Events

Questions 1–4: Passage Map

Topic: Flower arrangement
Scope: How to make it—materials & directions
Purpose: Explain step-by-step

1. **(A) at the 4:00 position.** Reread the steps looking for "third-longest stem" or look at your notes. The third-longest stem should be in the 4:00 position, which matches answer choice **(A)**. All other answer choices refer to other elements of the arrangement.

2. **(C) adding water to the dish.** Rereading the steps or using your notes, look for the first step. In the instructions, the key word "first" identifies this step, which is to add water to the dish. Choice (A) is the second step, (B) is the last, and (D) is the third.

3. **(C) pine, chrysanthemum, bamboo, iris** Because the directions state that stems are placed in decreasing order of their length, identify the longest as the first to be placed, which is pine. Now check the answer choices and eliminate any that do not start with pine. Only (A) and (C) are left. The next-longest item is the chrysanthemum, making choice **(C)** correct. All other answers are out of sequence, and choice (B) is completely backward, from shortest to longest.

4. **(A) in any place.** According to the directions, the third-longest stem (that is, the shortest) is the last stem to be placed in a specific position; after that, the florist can arrange any other plant materials in "any position that pleases you."

Questions 5–8: Passage Map

Topic: GG Bridge
Scope: When built, length, usage
Purpose: Inform

5. **(B) in a car.** According to the passage, pedestrians can cross the bridge only until 6:00 PST, but cars can cross at any time. Thus, a person crossing the bridge at 8:00 PM PST would need to be in a car. Choices (A) and (C) are incorrect because electric scooters and skateboards are never allowed on the bridge, and choice (D) is incorrect because pedestrians cannot walk across the bridge after 6:00 PST.

6. **(D) 1964.** The stimulus states that the Golden Gate bridge lost its title as the longest suspension bridge "when the Verrazano-Narrows bridge was built in New York in 1964," which matches choice **(D)**. All other dates are in the wrong decades.

7. **(D) 200,000** When the bridge opened to pedestrians on May 27, only one person was allowed to cross, but as the passage states, the next day, May 28, 200,000 people walked over the bridge. This matches answer choice **(D)**. Choice (A) gives the number of people who walked the bridge on opening day, choice (B) is the length of the bridge, and choice (C) is the number of vehicles that cross the bridge each day.

8. **(D) under construction.** The stimulus states that the bridge "was started in 1933 and finished in 1937," meaning that in 1936 it must still have been under construction. All other answers are incorrect use of details from the stimulus.

9. **(B)** The question asks you to identify a true statement about the results of arranging numbered shapes according to a set of instructions. Work step-by-step. The first four steps have you create 4 × 4 squares by arranging certain numbered squares from least to greatest in a clockwise direction.

1.

2	4
8	6

2.

1	3
7	5

3.

10	12
16	14

4.

9	11
15	13

While the previous steps had you arrange numbered squares *clockwise* to make 4 × 4 squares, step 5 has you arrange the 4 × 4 squares created in steps 1–4 *counter-clockwise*. So the 4 × 4 square containing the largest single number, 16, is at the upper left. Of the remaining 4 × 4 squares, the one containing the largest number is the one with 15, and it goes below the 4 × 4 square containing 16. The next 4 × 4 square, containing 8, goes to the right of that. And the final 4 × 4 square, whose largest number is 7, goes at the top right.

10	12	1	3
16	14	7	5
9	11	2	4
15	13	8	6

Mathematics Answers and Explanations

Chapter 1: Arithmetic and Algebra

Lesson 1: Arithmetic

1. **(C) $\frac{8}{25}$, 32%** You are asked to convert a decimal to a fraction and percent. To convert 0.32 to a fraction, note that the last digit, 2, is in the hundredths column, so write $\frac{32}{100}$. Reduce to lowest terms: $\frac{32}{100} = \frac{8}{25}$. To convert 0.32 to a percent, move the decimal point two places to the right and add a percent symbol: 32%. Check your work: confirm the simplification step and decimal placement.

2. **(C) 40** You are asked for the least common multiple (LCM) of three integers. Some multiples of 4 are 4, 8, 12, 16, 20, 24, 28, 32, 36, 40, 44. Some multiples of 8 are 6, 16, 24, 36, 40, 48. Some multiples of 10 are 10, 20, 30, 40, 50. The LCM of 4, 8, and 10 is 40—that's the smallest multiple they have in common.

3. **(B) $\frac{1}{4}, \frac{3}{8}, \frac{2}{5}$** You are asked to order the given fractions from least to greatest. To order the fractions, compare them in pairs using the X method. Comparing $\frac{3}{8}$ and $\frac{2}{5}$, you get $3 \times 5 = 15$ and $2 \times 8 = 16$. So $\frac{3}{8} < \frac{2}{5}$. Eliminate choice (A).

Comparing $\frac{3}{8}$ and $\frac{1}{4}$, you get $3 \times 4 = 12$ and $1 \times 8 = 8$. So $\frac{3}{8} > \frac{1}{4}$. The correct order is $\frac{1}{4}, \frac{3}{8}, \frac{2}{5}$. Alternatively, you could have converted $\frac{1}{4}$ to $\frac{2}{8}$ to make that comparison.

Double-check that you ranked the fractions from least to greatest. Choice (D) ranks them from greatest to least.

4. **(B) $2\frac{5}{24}$** Convert the mixed number to an improper fraction: $1\frac{5}{8} = \frac{(1 \times 8) + 5}{8} = \frac{8 + 5}{8} = \frac{13}{8}$. Find a common denominator for $\frac{13}{8}$ and $\frac{7}{12}$. The LCM of 8 and 12 is 24. Once you have converted each fraction, you can add

$\frac{13}{8} + \frac{7}{12} = \frac{13 \times 3}{8 \times 3} + \frac{7 \times 2}{12 \times 2} = \frac{39}{24} + \frac{14}{24} = \frac{53}{24}$. Now convert $\frac{53}{24}$ to a mixed number. When you divide 53 by 24, you get 2 with a remainder of 5. So, $\frac{53}{24} = 2\frac{5}{24}$.

5. **(D) 279** You are asked the value of an expression. Solve using PEMDAS. Becaue there are no exponents or parentheses, take care of division and multiplication first:

Multiplication/division: $81 + 12 - 18 + 204$
Addition/subtraction: $93 - 18 + 204$
$$75 + 204$$
$$279$$

6. **(C) 50** You are asked the value of an expression. Solve using PEMDAS.

Parentheses: $8 + 7 \times 6$
Multiplication/division: $8 + 42$
Addition/subtraction: 50

Lesson 2: Algebra

1. **(A) 7** The question asks you to solve for x. Use inverse operations. First, subtract 16 from both sides to yield $2x = 14$. Next, divide both sides by 2 to yield $x = 7$.

2. **(C) $14y + 70$** The question asks you to simplify, so combine like terms. Note that when you add the variable terms $5y + 9y = 14y$, you can quickly eliminate two of the answer choices, (A) and (B). Next, add $-11 + 81 = 70$. Note that this is the same as subtracting 11 from 81: $81 - 11 = 70$. Finally, add the terms: $14y + 70$. These are unlike terms, so the expression cannot be further simplified.

3. **(C) 3** The question asks you to solve for b. First, add 21 to both sides to yield $10b = 30$. Next, divide both sides by 10 to yield $b = 3$.

4. **(D) $56x + 4$** The question asks you to add the expressions, so combine like terms. Note that when you add the variable terms $44x + 12x = 56x$, you can quickly eliminate two of the answer choices, (A) and (B). Next, add: $-1 + 5 = 4$. Finally, add the unlike terms: $56x + 4$.

5. **(D) 10** The question asks you to solve for a. First, to cancel the division on the left side, multiply both sides by 2 to yield $5a = 2(2a + 5)$. Next, simplify on the right side: $5a = 4a + 10$. Finally, subtract $4a$ from both sides to yield $a = 10$.

Lesson 3: Solving Word Problems

1. **(C) $15.75** This question gives you information about the cost of different food items and asks for the total spent on lunch. To find a total, add the individual amounts. Because they "both" get a soda, first multiply the $1.50 for the soda by 2: $1.50 \times 2 = 3.00. Then add the sandwich and mac 'n' cheese: $3.00 + $8.00 + 4.75 = 15.75. You can check your work by subtracting each food item from the total: $15.75 − $8.00 − $4.75 − $1.50 − $1.50 = 0.

2. **(B) $257.50** You're given information about Jamal's monthly income and his expenses, and you're asked how much he will save each month. Find the money left over after expenses by subtracting from the total: $2,875 − $2,360 = $515. He will save only half of that, so divide by 2: $515 ÷ 2 = $257.50. Check your work by performing the calculations in reverse: double $257.50 and add it to $2,360 to get $2,875.

3. **(A) 5** This word problem presents information about the number of students who have chosen different art projects and the number of crayons available. It asks you to calculate how many crayons the teacher gives "each student" if she distributes them "equally." Divide the total number of crayons, 60, by the total number of students ($3 + 9 = 12$): $60 ÷ 12 = 5$. Check your work by reversing the calculations: Does 12 students times 5 crayons each equal 60 crayons? Yes, it does.

4. **(D) 60** This word problem gives you information about Tyler's strawberry growing: how many bales of straw to grow a pallet of strawberries and how much profit he makes on six pallets. You need to find the number of bales of straw it takes to earn a $400 profit. First, divide Tyler's total profit by his profit per six pallets: $400 ÷ $80 = 5$. He needs to sell six pallets five times to earn $400 profit; in other words, he needs to sell $6 \times 5 = 30$ pallets. Then he needs two bales of straw per pallet, so multiply 30 pallets by 2 bales to get the total bales needed: $30 \times 2 = 60$ bales of straw.

5. **(B) 35 minutes** You are told the distance Kaitlyn travels to work and her different speeds in the morning and the afternoon. The amount of distance traveled equals the speed of travel multiplied by the time spent traveling. Translate this into the formula distance = rate × time. To calculate her travel time, rearrange the formula: $\text{time} = \dfrac{\text{distance}}{\text{rate}}$. Because she travels at different rates, perform the calculation twice. Morning: $\dfrac{10 \text{ miles}}{40 \text{ mph}} = \dfrac{1}{4}$ hours = 15 minutes. Afternoon: $\dfrac{10 \text{ miles}}{30 \text{ mph}} = \dfrac{1}{3}$ hours = 20 minutes. Then add the times to get the total: 15 minutes + 20 minutes = 35 minutes.

6. **(B) 24** First, calculate how much money the therapist would earn at Clinic A. Translate "$25 per patient treated" into $25 per patient × 30 patients = $750. Then translate "plus a flat weekly salary of $200" into $750 + $200 = $950. This is the total weekly income at Clinic A. If the total weekly income at Clinic B equaled this amount, the equation would be $40 × B = $950, where B is the number of patients seen. Find B: $950 ÷ $40 per patient = 23.75 patients. You want the therapist's income at Clinic B to exceed that at Clinic A, so he needs to see more than 23.75 patients. Because there can't be partial patients (and all the answers, thankfully, are whole numbers), round up to the nearest whole number. The minimum number of patients at Clinic B necessary to earn more than $950 is 24.

7. **(D) $45 \leq n \leq 90$** This question presents a scenario about varying rates of cars passing through a light, and the answer choices are inequalities. You need to calculate the range of possible numbers of cars that can pass in 15 minutes. Start by calculating how many cars can pass in a minute at the minimum rate: 60 seconds ÷ 10 seconds per car = 6 cars per minute. Now calculate how many can pass at the maximum rate: 60 seconds ÷ 20 seconds per car = 3 cars per minute. (Note that the "in between" rate of one car every 15 seconds is irrelevant to your calculations, because you only need to find the minimum and maximum rates.) Once you've calculated the minimum and maximum number of cars per minute, multiply each quantity by 15 minutes: 3 cars per minute × 15 minutes = 45 cars; 6 cars per minute × 15 minutes 90 cars. Thus, 45 is the minimum number of cars that will pass, and 90 is the maximum. n is greater than or equal to 45 and less than or equal to 90.

8. **(D) 40** Because the vegetable garden uses one-fourth of 36 gallons, translate that into $\dfrac{1}{4} \times 36 = 9$, so 9 gallons are applied to the vegetables. Thus, the filter processes 9 gallons of water per day. The question says the filter needs replacement after 360 gallons, so divide this amount by the gallons per day to find the number of days the filter will last before it has to be replaced: 360 gallons ÷ 9 gallons per day = 40 days.

Lesson 4: Ratios, Percentages, and Proportions

1. **(C) 20% increase** The question states that the value of the investment first dropped by 20% but then increased by 50% from the lowered value and asks for the overall percent change. Because no specific values are given and this question is about percentages, pick 100 as the starting value of Juanita's investment. The 20% drop then would have been $\frac{20}{100} \times 100 = 20$. Subtract 20 from 100 to determine the reduced value of 80. The 50% increase was based on this reduced value: $\frac{50}{100} \times 80 = \frac{1}{2} \times 80 = 40$. Add this increase of 40 to 80 to obtain a final value of 120. At this point, you know the value of the investment went up (from 100 to 120), so eliminate choices (A) and (B). Finally, use the formula for percentage change, subtracting the starting value from the new value and setting that over 100: $\frac{120 - 100}{100} = \frac{20}{100} = 20\%$. Choice (D) is a trap answer because it equals $50 - 20$, but the 50% increase was based on a lower value. Check your logic and calculations.

2. **(B) 400** The question asks you to determine the amount that 60 would be 15% of. Percentage problems with an unknown value can be set up as a proportion: $\frac{15}{100} = \frac{60}{x}$. Cross multiply to obtain $15x = 6000$. To avoid more difficult long division, tackle this in two steps. Both sides of the equation are divisible by 3, so $5x = 2000$. Now divide both sides by 5 to get $x = 400$. Verify your logic in setting up the proportion and check your math.

3. **(A) 5 bandages and 4 swabs** The question lists the desired ratio of three items and the current inventory of those items, and it asks how many of what two types of supplies must be added to bring the inventory ratio into line. The requirement to add to the stock of only two items is a clue as to how to solve this problem. By comparing the current inventory of each item to the specified ratio, you can determine which of the three supplies will not need to be augmented. There are 6 units of ointment and its part of the ratio is 2, so the "multiplier" for that supply is $6 \div 2 = 3$. For the bandages, the multiplier is $10 \div 5 = 2$, so some bandages will need to be added. The multiplier for swabs is $20 \div 8 = 2.5$, so some swabs will need to be added as well. To bring the multiplier for bandages up to 3 to "match" the multiplier for ointment, there should be $3 \times 5 = 15$ in inventory, which would require adding 5 more to the current inventory of 10. There need to be $3 \times 8 = 24$ swabs,

a quantity that is obtained by adding 4 swabs to the current inventory of 20. The correct answer is **(A)**. Another way to solve this problem would be to try each answer choice and calculate the resulting ratio until you find the correct answer. Check your answer to be certain it is correct: divide each term of 6:15:24 by 3 to get the desired inventory ratio, 2:5:8.

4. **(D) 8** The question provides the scale proportionality of a drawing and the measured length of a hallway on that plan. You are asked to determine how many 8-foot pieces of molding are needed for *both* sides of that hallway. To determine the actual length of the hallway, set up a proportion based on the scale of the drawing: $\frac{\frac{1}{4} \text{ in.}}{1 \text{ ft}} = \frac{7\frac{3}{4} \text{ in.}}{x \text{ ft}}$. (Its all right to mix inches and feet because both ratios have inches in the numerator and feet in the denominator.) Cross multiply to get $\frac{1}{4}x = 7\frac{3}{4}(1) = \frac{31}{4}$. Now you can multiply both sides of that equation by 4 to get $x = 31$ feet. The question states that the molding is being installed on *both* sides of the hallway, so $2 \times 31 = 62$ feet are needed. The molding is purchased in 8-foot pieces. Because 8 pieces total 64 feet in length and 7 pieces would leave you short, at only 56 feet in length, 8 is the number that must be bought. Choice (A), 4 pieces, is a trap answer because that is the number of pieces needed for *one* side of the hallway. Verify that you answered the question that was asked, that you set up the proportion properly, and that your calculations are accurate.

5. **(D) $\frac{0.2 \text{ cc}}{\text{minute}}$** The question provides the amounts of fluid in an IV bag at two different times. This particular solution has a concentration of 5% medication, and the question asks for the unit rate at which the medication is dispensed. First, determine the drip rate of the total solution: $\frac{780 \text{ cc} - 300 \text{ cc}}{(10 - 8) \text{ hours}} = \frac{480 \text{ cc}}{2 \text{ hours}} = 240 \frac{\text{cc}}{\text{hour}}$. Because only 5% of the solution is medication, that would be $0.05 \times 240 = 12$ cc of medication per hour. Unfortunately, none of the answer choices match that delivery rate. Choice (A) is a trap answer; this is the delivery rate of the solution rather than the medication. Also, be careful of choice (B): this is mathematically correct, but *unit* rates are stated with a denominator of 1. Both of the remaining choices are expressed as unit rates per minute, so divide the hourly rate by 60 to obtain the rate per minute: $12 \frac{\text{cc}}{\text{hour}} \div \frac{60 \text{ minutes}}{1 \text{ hour}} = 12 \frac{\text{cc}}{\text{hour}} \times \frac{1 \text{ hour}}{60 \text{ minutes}} = 0.2 \frac{\text{cc}}{\text{minute}}$. Double-check that you used the correct values from the question and that your logic and calculations are correct.

Lesson 5: Estimating and Rounding

1. **(B) 3** The question asks you to convert a measurement from cubic centimeters to the nearest liter. The answer choices are all displayed as whole numbers. Because a liter is defined as 1000 cubic centimeters, divide 2753 by 1000. Do this by moving the decimal point 3 places to the left to get 2.753. Round this result to the nearest liter by looking at the first digit to the right of the decimal point. Because this number is 7, round up to 3 liters.

2. **(B) 378** A quick glance at the answer choices reveals that they are far enough apart that estimating will be an efficient approach. Round the given numbers to get $(60 - 40) \times (40 - 20)$. So, $20 \times 20 = 400$. The answer choice closest to 400 is **(B)**, 378.

3. **(C) 1056 mL** The question provides the hourly rate of leakage from a faucet and asks how much water would be lost over 2 days. A quick glance at the answer choices shows that they are widely spaced, so you can estimate the correct answer. Convert days to hours to match the units in the drip rate:
$2 \text{ days} \times \dfrac{24 \text{ hrs}}{\text{day}} = 48 \text{ hrs}.$ Round 48 up to 50 and the drip rate down from 22 to 20. Because one number was rounded up and one down, it will be safe to multiply to get an estimate:
$20 \dfrac{\text{mL}}{\text{hr}} \times 50 \text{ hrs} = 1000 \text{ mL}.$ Scanning the answer choices, only **(C)**, 1056 mL, is close to this estimate.

4. **(C) 12** The problem provides information about the number of cookies per case and the average breakage rate, and it asks for the expected number of broken cookies per case. This is a percentage rate problem that can be solved by estimating because the answer will be rounded to a whole number and the answer choices are quite spread out. The breakage rate is given as a percentage, so set up a proportion, with 30×24 representing the total number of cookies in a case:
$\dfrac{1.72}{100} = \dfrac{x}{30 \times 24}.$ To simplify the calculations, round 24 down to 20 and 1.72 up to 2: $\dfrac{2}{100} = \dfrac{x}{30 \times 20} = \dfrac{x}{600}.$ Cross multiply to get $100x = 1200$ and $x = 12$. The estimate of 12 exactly equals correct answer **(C)**.

Note that after cross multiplication, the 24, 30, and 1.72 were all multiplied together. Because the amount of rounding was significant (1.72 up to 2 accounts for just over a 15% increase, and 24 down to 20 is a little over a 15% decrease), it's important that they were rounded in opposite directions. In fact, even if there were 25 packages in a case, it would still be more accurate to round down than up, despite the "5 and up" rule. Consider the cumulative effect of rounding when adding or multiplying many numbers together and break the rules when necessary.

5. **(A) 1161** The question asks for the value of the product of two 2-digit numbers. The estimated value of this expression is $30 \times 40 = 1200$. Given the closely spaced answer choices, that estimate is of no value. However, there is another shortcut that can occasionally be used with multiplication questions: the last-digit test. If you were to actually multiply 27 by 43, you would start with $7 \times 3 = 21$, and the last digit of the product would be 1. Before plodding through the rest of the multiplication process, check the answer choices to see if this tidbit of information is helpful. Sure enough, only choice **(A)** ends with 1, so that has to be the correct answer.

Science Answers and Explanations

Chapter 1: Human Anatomy and Physiology

Lesson 1: Human Anatomy and Physiology: An Overview

1. **(B) Lysosomes** Macrophages will need extra organelles whose primary function is to break down cellular waste, so macrophages will have more lysosomes.

2. **(A) Urinary** The function of the urinary system is to filter the blood and eliminate waste products. Urine is named after its main component, urea, which is produced in the liver.

3. **(D) transverse** The transverse plane divides the body into top (superior) and bottom (inferior) halves.

Lesson 2: The Skeletal System

1. **(A) Osteoblast** Osteoporosis is caused by a demineralization of bone. Treatment would increase the activity, or *upregulate*, the activity of bone-building cells, osteoblasts.

2. **(B) Humerus** The humerus is a long bone found in the upper arm. Carpals, located in the wrist, are short bones. The vertebrae are irregular bones, and the pelvis is a flat bone.

Lesson 3: The Neuromuscular System

1. **(A) an afferent neuron.** Messages transmitted to the brain are sent via sensory neurons, also called afferent neurons. Efferent neurons and motor neurons refer to the same type of nerve, which relays messages from the brain back to the musculature. The brain stem sends and receives messages related to critical involuntary functions.

2. **(B) difficulty walking.** The cerebellum is the part of the brain involved in motor control and muscle coordination. Speech and short-term memory would be affected by damage to the frontal lobe of the cerebrum, whereas damage to the brain stem would result in life-threatening injuries to critical body functions such as heartbeat and respiration.

3. **(D) Muscle fibers contract in an all-or-none fashion.** Even when a person is at rest, vital muscular contractions involving smooth muscle are still occurring. Muscle contraction is activated by actin and myosin; myelin is the insulation surrounding axons. Sensory neurons carry signals from the muscle to the brain; motor neurons stimulate muscle tissue to contract.

Lesson 4: The Cardiovascular System

1. **(D) Tricuspid** The tricuspid valve separates the right atrium from the right ventricle. The aortic valve prevents blood from backflowing from the aorta into the left ventricle. The terms *bicuspid valve* and *mitral valve* both refer to the valve that separates the left atrium from the left ventricle.

2. **(C) Left ventricle - aorta - capillaries - vena cava - right ventricle** From the left ventricle, blood flows through the circuit system to the aorta, then through the arteries, arterioles, and capillaries, and then returns to the heart via venules, veins, and the vena cava, where it enters the right atrium. It flows through the pulmonary circuit from the right atrium to the right ventricle, then through the pulmonary artery to the lungs, returning to the left atrium via the pulmonary vein.

3. **(A) Platelets** Hemoglobin is responsible for binding oxygen in the red blood cell. Lymph is the fluid of the open circulatory system that removes waste products from the tissues. Antibodies are plasma proteins that work with the immune system to remove foreign pathogens.

English and Language Usage Answers and Explanations

Chapter 1: Spelling, Punctuation, and Sentence Structure

Lesson 1: Spelling

1. **(C) Wierd** "Weird" is an exception to the "*i* before *e*" rule.

2. **(D) injurious** The root word, "injury," ends in a *y* that is preceded by a consonant, so the REBS rule to follow is "Change the *y* to *i* and add the suffix."

3. **(A) frolicked** The root word, "frolic," ends in a *c*, so the REBS rule to follow is "Add a *k* when adding a suffix beginning with *e, i,* or *y*."

4. **(B) principal/principles.** "Principal," used here as an adjective modifying "reason," means "primary," and "principle" is a noun that means "guiding rule." Note that when *principal* is used as a noun, it refers either to the leader of a school or to an amount of money that is invested to earn interest.

Lesson 2: Punctuation

1. **(C) Although I am an experienced hiker, I was not prepared for the rocky terrain.** Choice (A) is a simple sentence, and a comma is missing after the introductory prepositional phrase. Choice (B) is an incorrectly punctuated compound sentence—a semicolon is missing before "however." Because it is both the wrong sentence structure and incorrectly punctuated, eliminate. Choice (D) is a complex sentence, but it incorrectly offsets the subordinate clause with a comma. In this choice, the comma is incorrect since the subordinate clause appears after the independent clause. Choice **(C)** is a correctly punctuated complex sentence.

2. **(B) "We must all do our part," she said, "even when doing so is difficult."** When a direct quote is interrupted by a reference to the speaker, the first half of the quote should end in a comma, and the second half should be introduced with a comma.

3. **(D) Because the weather forecast predicted storms, we decided to postpone our vacation until next month.** "Because the weather forecast predicted storms" is a subordinate clause and must be followed by a comma.

4. **(B) ;** The sentence is made up of two independent clauses. When two independent clauses need to be connected in a sentence and no conjunction is present, a semicolon should be placed between the two clauses.

Lesson 3: Sentence Structure

1. **(A) Working** The independent clause is "Working hard is important," because this could stand alone as a complete sentence. "Working" is the subject—the thing that "is important." This is an example of a verb form having *-ing* added and being used as a noun (it's called a *gerund*). "Important" is a complement. The other words are in the dependent clause. Note that in a complex sentence like this one, the subject of the independent clause is also the subject of the sentence.

2. **(C) his** A pronoun is a word that is used instead of a noun. "His" is the pronoun that refers back to the noun "Bob."

3. **(A) Because the book was confusing, Sarah stopped reading it, so now she needs something new to read.** This is the only sentence to incorporate two independent clauses and one or more dependent clauses. The independent clauses are "Sarah stopped reading the book" and "so now she needs something new to read."

4. **(D) story** The direct object is a person or thing that receives the action of the verb. The story (the direct object) is being told to me (the indirect object).

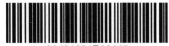

36481031R00115

Made in the USA
Middletown, DE
02 November 2016